VITILIGO AND OTHER PIGMENTARY DISORDERS

VITILIGO AND OTHER PIGMENTARY DISORDERS

Lalit Kumar Gupta
MD (AIIMS, N. Delhi), FAAD
Senior Professor
Department of Dermatology
RNT Medical College, Udaipur (Raj), India

Nidheesh Agarwal
MD
Assistant Professor
Department of Dermatology
Geetanjali Medical College, Udaipur (Raj), India

PEEPEE
PUBLISHERS AND DISTRIBUTORS (P) LTD.

VITILIGO AND OTHER PIGMENTARY DISORDERS

Published by
Pawaninder P. Vij and Anupam Vij
Peepee Publishers and Distributors (P) Ltd.
Head Office: 160, Shakti Vihar, Pitam Pura
Delhi-110034 (India)

Correspondence Address:
7/31, First Floor, Ansari Road
Daryaganj, New Delhi-110002 (India)
Ph: 65195868, 23246245, 9811156083
e-mail: peepee160@yahoo.co.in, peepee160@rediffmail.com
peepee160@gmail.com
Website: www.peepeepub.com

First Edition: 2016

ISBN: 978-81-8445-190-0

Dedicated to

Our Patients, Parents and Teachers

Our Wives: Anjana and Sunanda

Our Children: Sujay and Vartika

FOREWORD

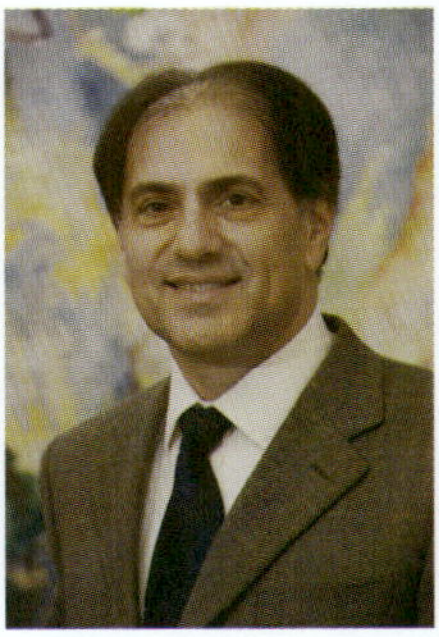

It gives me immense pleasure to introduce the book **"Vitiligo and Other Pigmentary Disorders"** by Prof. Lalit Gupta and Prof Nidheesh Agarwal. Vitiligo is a common depigmentary disease of great cosmetic concern and devastating psycho-social consequences, particularly in type IV and type V skin. Melasma is another common hyper-pigmentary problem seen both in fair as well as dark skin.

This book is an attempt by the authors to familiarize primary care physicians, internists and dermatologists about a wide variety of pigmentary diseases and provide them with a systematic approach in diagnosis and effective management of these conditions. Emphasis has been laid on vitiligo and melasma (as they are the most commonly encountered problems) and other disorders have been discussed with a focus on practically useful points in diagnosis and management. The authors have used their vast experience in writing this concise yet comprehensive account on pigmentary diseases seen in the skin of dark. Text is written in simple, point-wise, bulleted format and is backed up with excellent quality photographs, tables and flowcharts to make the comprehension easy.

I hope that this crisp and informative textbook **"Vitiligo and Other Pigmentary Disorders"** will help readers in better managing their patients with pigmentary disorders, mitigating their sufferings.

Professor Thomas Ruzicka
Chairman
Department of Dermatology and Allergy
Ludwig Maximilian University of Munich, Germany

PREFACE

" There is only one good, knowledge, and one evil, ignorance."

—Socrates, Greek Philosopher (470 BC-399 BC)

Pigmentary disorders of skin, though seemingly benign and not life threatening, have a profound impact on the quality of life of patients. Besides cosmetic concern, these diseases cause a great deal of social stigma and tremendous psychological stress leading to anxiety, depression, fear of rejection, low self esteem and even suicidal tendencies. A large part of clinical practice of dermatologists and general practitioners comprises managing patients with these disorders.

"**Vitiligo and Other Pigmentary Disorders**" is an attempt by authors to familiarize the clinicians with common as well as not so common pigmentary diseases seen in India. Dermatology residents, internists and primary care physicians will particularly benefit from this short textbook due to its simple, concise and easy to understand text backed up with excellent quality clinical photographs. The emphasis is laid on the two most commonly encountered conditions—vitiligo and melasma while for others most practical diagnostic and therapeutic tips are included. Exhaustive theoretical details are deliberately omitted to maintain the brevity of text and for readers seeking more information, "Suggested Readings" has been included at the end of each chapter.

We hope that this short textbook on **"Vitiligo and Other Pigmentary Disorders"** will benefit the readers in better managing their patients with pigmentary diseases and help mitigate their sufferings.

LALIT KUMAR GUPTA
NIDHEESH AGARWAL

ACKNOWLEDGEMENTS

We gratefully acknowledge the contribution of following in providing the clinical pictures:

Miss Vartika Gupta: Fig. 1.1

Dr Khushboo Gupta: Fig. 3.2

Dr Sanjay Rathi: Fig. 3.15, 3.16 (a,b,c)

Dr Paschal D'Souza, Dr Akhilesh Shukla and Dr Mayank Kaushik: Fig. 5.1, 5.7, 5.27

Dr Astha Sharma: Fig. 5.29

Dr Swati Tripathi: Fig. 2.8, 5.7

Our special gratitude to the directors of Peepee Publishers and Distributors Pvt. Ltd., Pawaninder P Vij and Anupam Vij for their continued cooperation in enabling this project seeing the light of the day.

CONTRIBUTORS

Lalit Kumar Gupta
MD (AIIMS, N. Delhi), FAAD
Senior Professsor
Department of Dermatology
RNT Medical College, Udaipur (Raj), India

Ashok Kumar Khare, MD
Senior Professor and Head
Department of Dermatology
RNT Medical College, Udaipur (Raj), India

Nidheesh Agarwal, MD
Assistant Professor
Department of Dermatology
Geetanjali Medical College, Udaipur (Raj), India

Manisha Balai, MD
Assistant Professor
Department of Dermatology
RNT Medical College, Udaipur (Raj), India

Urvashi Goyal
MD Scholar
Department of Dermatology
RNT Medical College, Udaipur (Raj), India

Chesta Agrawal
MD Scholar
Department of Dermatology
RNT Medical College, Udaipur (Raj), India

CONTENTS

1 FUNDAMENTALS OF SKIN COLOR AND MELANOGENESIS

Lalit K Gupta, Nidheesh Agarwal

Chapter At A Glance

- **Melanin is the main pigment responsible for color of skin.**
- **Melanocyte number does not differ in different races, while its activity does.**
- **In melanocytes, melanin is synthesized inside the melanosomes with the help of tyrosinase enzyme and transferred to keratinocytes.**
- **One melanocyte associates with 36 keratinocytes forming an "epidermal melanin unit".**
- **Ultraviolet (UV) radiation is the main stimulus for melanogenesis.**
- **The main function of melanin is to protect skin from harmful UV rays.**

- Normal skin color is due to the presence of chromophores, the most important of which is melanin, synthesized by melanocytes (melanogenesis).
- Melanocytes are dendritic cells derived from neural crest and are mainly present in basal layer of epidermis, hair bulb, outer root sheath of hair follicles, eyes, cochlea, adrenals and meninges.
- Melanin is synthesized in the organelles called melanosomes and then transferred to keratinocytes. Keratinocytes normally contain more melanin than melanocytes. There is approximately

one melanocyte per 5 or 6 basal keratinocytes. One melanocyte generally donates melanosomes to around 36 keratinocytes and this association forms the *epidermal melanin unit* (Fig.1.1).

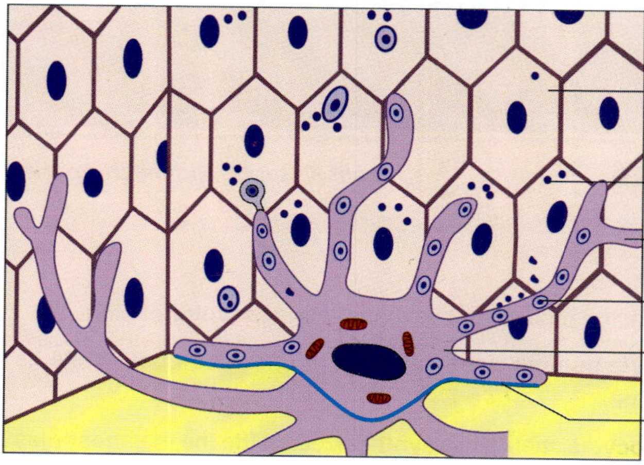

Fig. 1.1: Epidermal melanin unit

- Melanocyte density ranges from approximately 550 to >1200 per mm^2 with highest concentration found in genitals and face. It is about two fold higher in exposed than non-exposed skin. A reduction in number of melanocytes occurs with age by 6-8% per decade.
- Two types of melanin occur in skin
  - **Eumelanin:** Dark brown/black, insoluble.
  - **Pheomelanin:** Pale red or yellow, sulfur containing, soluble.
- Racial and ethnic differences in skin color are mainly due to shape, size, distribution and degradation of melanosomes and not due to differences in the number of melanocytes.
- Melanins are indole derivatives of 3,4 dihydroxyphenylalanine (DOPA) and are formed in melanosomes through a series of oxidative steps (Fig.1.2). Tyrosinase is the main enzyme in melanin biosynthetic pathway.

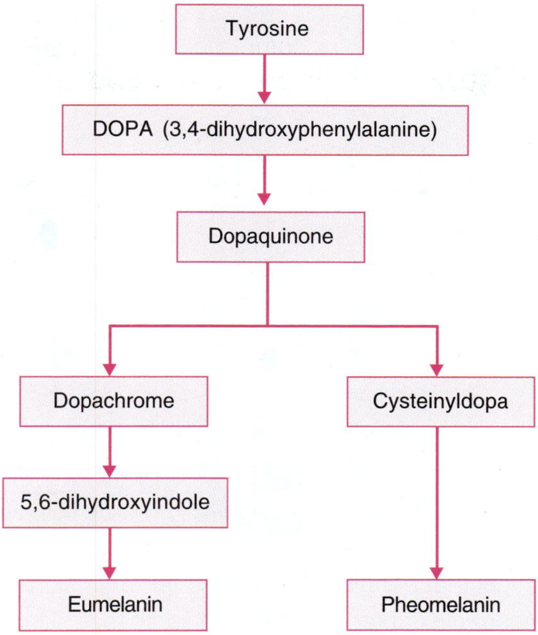

Fig. 1.2: Melanin biosynthesis in melanocytes

- The overall skin color of a person is determined by 2 factors
  - **Constitutive:** In the absence of sun and other influences.
  - **Facultative:** 'Tan' that results from sun exposure.
- Endocrine (mainly melanocyte stimulating hormone–MSH), paracrine and autocrine factors also control pigmentation.
- Based on the tolerance of skin to sun and tanning properties, 6 skin types have been described called Fitzpatrick skin types (Table 1.1). Indian skin represents 4/5 skin type.
- The main function of melanin is to protect the skin from harmful effects of ultraviolet radiation. This is evident from the fact that UV induced carcinoma occur with a higher frequency in fair skinned persons.

Table 1.1: Fitzpatrick's skin types

Skin phenotype	Sun sensitivity	Tanning ability
I	Very sensitive, burns very easily	No or little tan
II	Very sensitive, always burns	Minimal tan
III	Sensitive, burns moderately	Tan slowly (light brown)
IV	Moderate sensitivity, burns sometimes	Tan easily (brown)
V	Minimally sensitive, rarely burns	Tan dark brown
VI	Insensitive, never burns	Deeply pigmented (black)

- It is ironical that people with fair skin tan their skin to get darker while those with darker color tend to bleach their skin in an attempt to achieve fairness despite the fact that *"black is beautiful"* in terms of UV protective ability.
- Two basic patterns of pigmentary abnormalities are seen characterized by decreased pigmentation (hypopigmentary disorders) and increased pigmentation (hyperpigmentary disorders).
- Some common examples of hypopigmentary disorders include vitiligo, albinism, chemical leucoderma, infective conditions like pityriasis versicolor, leprosy, post kala azar dermal leishmaniasis (PKDL) and post-inflammatory hypopigmentation secondary to some disorders like lupus erythematosus, scleroderma, burns and scalds.
- Melasma is the most common hyperpigmentary disorder. The other conditions are freckles, lentigenes, Addison's disease, nutritional deficiency, medications and post-inflammatory hyper-pigmentation.

Suggested Readings

1. Bhat R; *Vitiligo and Disorders of Hypopigmentation*, In: Vishwanath V, editor, *IADVL's Concise Textbook of Dermatology*, 1st edn., Wiley-Blackwell 2012, pp. 221-29.

2. Khanna N; *Disorders of Pigmentation*, In: *Illustrated Synopsis of Dermatology and Sexually Transmitted Diseases,* 2nd edn., Elsevier 2008, pp. 125-37.

3. Park HY, Pongpudpunth M, Lee J, Yaar M; *Biology of Melanocytes*, In: Wolff K, Goldsmith LA, Katz SI, Gilchrest BA, Paller AS, Leffell DJ, editors, *Fitzpatrick's Dermatology in General Medicine*, 7th edn., Mc Graw Hill 2008, pp. 591-607.

2 VITILIGO

Nidheesh Agarwal, Lalit K Gupta

Chapter At A Glance

- Vitiligo is an acquired disease characterized by progressive loss of melanocytes.
- Vitiligo has significant psychosocial impact and is responsible for degradation of quality of life, especially in young Indian females.
- It is the most common hypopigmentary disorder.
- Etiopathogenesis is not very well understood, current evidence most strong for autoimmune etiology.
- Certain predisposing factors precipitate the disease in genetically susceptible individuals.
- May involve skin and mucosa; preferably affects naturally hyperpigmented regions of the body and trauma prone sites.
- Two main clinical types: Segmental and non-segmental vitiligo.
- Although many therapies exist, no cure for the disease has yet been found.
- Topical corticosteroids and "Narrow band ultraviolet B" (NB-UVB) are first line therapies for treatment of vitiligo.
- Facial lesions respond well to topical calcineurin inhibitors; acral lesions and those over bony prominences are the most resistant to any form of therapy.
- Surgical therapies may be useful when medical and light therapies fail.
- Counselling and camouflage form very important aspects of therapy.

HISTORICAL BACKGROUND AND INTRODUCTION

The word 'Vitiligo' is derived from 'Vitium' meaning defect or blemish, and was first used by Celsus in his medical classic 'De Medicina'. Ancient Indian medical texts refer to it by various names such as Kilasa, Sveta Khista, Charak and the disease was often confused with leprosy. Earliest references to vitiligo in ancient literature date back to 2200 BC. Vitiligo patients have suffered from social stigma since the ancient times, and have been forbidden to marry, mingle with others and attend places of worship, in different communities across the world.

Modern day synonyms and vernaculars are leukoderma, phulwari or simply 'white spot disease'. Vitiligo can be defined as an *acquired hypopigmentary disorder characterized by progressive loss of melanocytes*. The disease not only has cosmetic importance, but also has a tremendous psychosocial impact and deteriorates the quality of life, particularly in communities with darker skin types.

EPIDEMIOLOGY

Vitiligo is one of the most common cutaneous disorders. Although more common and cosmetically more concerning in pigmented skin, it can affect all racial and ethnic groups. The prevalence varies between geographical regions from 0.1% to 3% in different studies worldwide; 0.5-1% in most populations. India has the highest prevalence rates of vitiligo, ranging from 0.25% to 8.8%, with the state of Gujarat having the highest rate worldwide at 8.8%.There is no sex predilection. Girls develop the disease at an earlier age than boys, and are more likely to seek treatment. The onset is earlier in cases with positive family history, which ranges from 7.7% to 50%. Vitiligo can occur at any age, with approximately half the cases developing before 20 years of age. Childhood vitiligo has some distinct clinico-epidemiological features (Fig. 2.1).

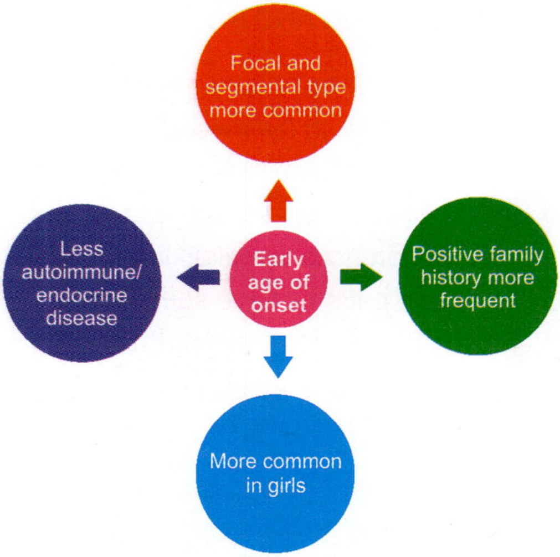

Fig. 2.1: Characteristics of childhood vitiligo

ETIOPATHOGENESIS

Vitiligo is a disease with unknown cause. Many etiologic hypotheses have been postulated (Fig. 2.2) but none explains all the aspects of vitiligo. Current understanding of the disease is that it represents not a single disease entity but a syndrome of heterogenous pathophysiological disorders presenting with depigmentation.

Genetic Hypothesis

Approximately 20-30% patients of vitiligo give a positive family history. It is presumed that vitiligo is inherited in a non-Mendelian, multifactorial, polygenic pattern with incomplete penetrance.

Autoimmune Hypothesis

Current evidence and global consensus point towards an autoimmune hypothesis. It is supported by the association of vitiligo with autoimmune disorders in various genetic association studies. Also, the cellular and humoral aberrations seen in vitiligo patients indicate an autoimmune etiology.

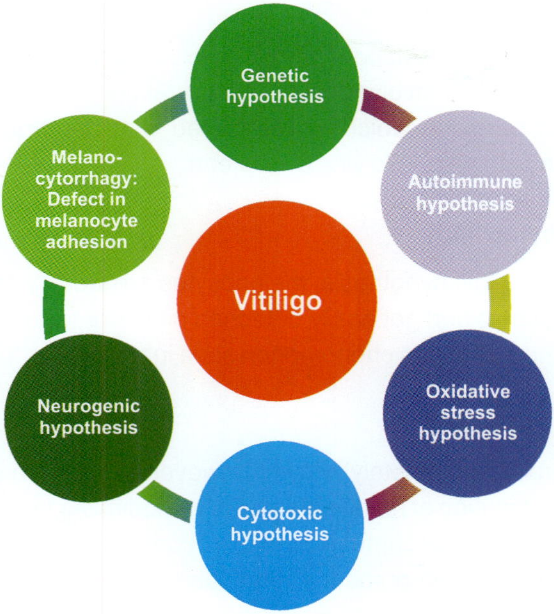

Fig. 2.2: Various hypothesis for etiopathogenesis of vitiligo

Neurogenic Hypothesis

Vitiligo in some patients is segmental along the distribution of nerves and is associated with neuronal dysregulation. This dysregulation may be local, in the form of increased neurotransmitter release (such as neuropeptide Y and norepinephrine) which may be directly or indirectly cytotoxic to cells. Systemic neuronal dysregulation (during periods of stress) has also been known to be a predisposing factor for vitiligo.

Cytotoxic Hypothesis

Various toxic substances, both environmental and endogenous, may accumulate and damage melanocytes in genetically susceptible individuals. Phenols and quinones are the suspected culprits.

Oxidative Stress Hypothesis

Vitiligo patients have abnormally low levels of catalase enzyme, both in involved and uninvolved skin. This correlates with high levels of hydrogen peroxide which is associated with deranged melanin synthesis pathways involving 6-biopterin.

Melanocytorrhagy

According to this hypothesis, melanocytes are weakly anchored in vitiligo patients and get easily detached on minor friction. This may explain the Koebner's phenomenon seen in vitiligo.

Predisposing Factors

These are not completely known, however it has been suggested that a combination of modifiable and non-modifiable factors such as genotype, stress, accumulation of toxic compounds, autoimmunity, altered cellular environment and melanocyte migration, infections and mutations converge to cause the disease (Fig. 2.3).

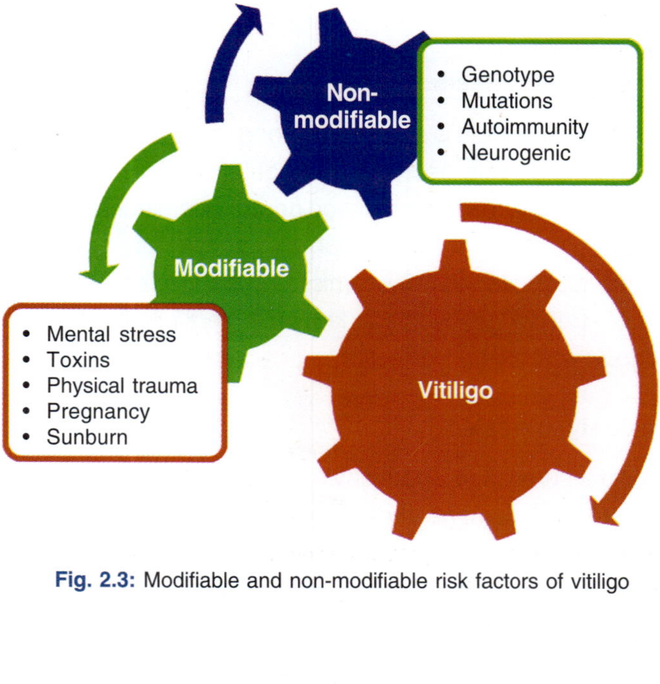

Fig. 2.3: Modifiable and non-modifiable risk factors of vitiligo

CLINICAL FEATURES

- Vitiligo typically presents as asymptomatic, chalky white, well demarcated depigmented macular lesions.
- The margins are usually convex but may be scalloped (Fig. 2.4), and get accentuated under Wood's light.
- The lesions are more common on normally hyperpigmented areas of the body such as face (especially periocular and perioral regions), axillae, groins, genitalia and areolae (Figs. 2.4 to 2.8). The distribution of lesions forms the basis of classification of vitiligo.

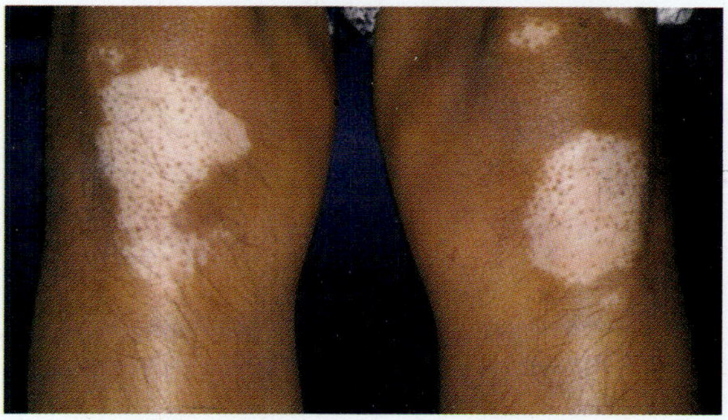

Fig. 2.4: Lesions on trauma prone sites (knees) in a child with perifollicular repigmentation. Also note the scalloped borders of the lesions

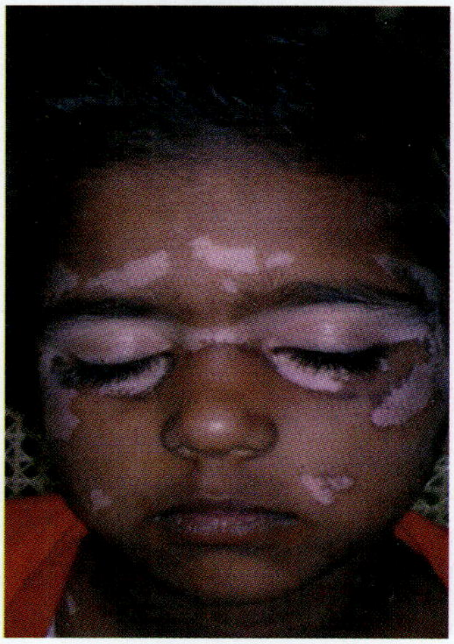

Fig. 2.5: Lesions over face, predominantly periocular. Note the hyperpigmentation at the periphery of the lesions

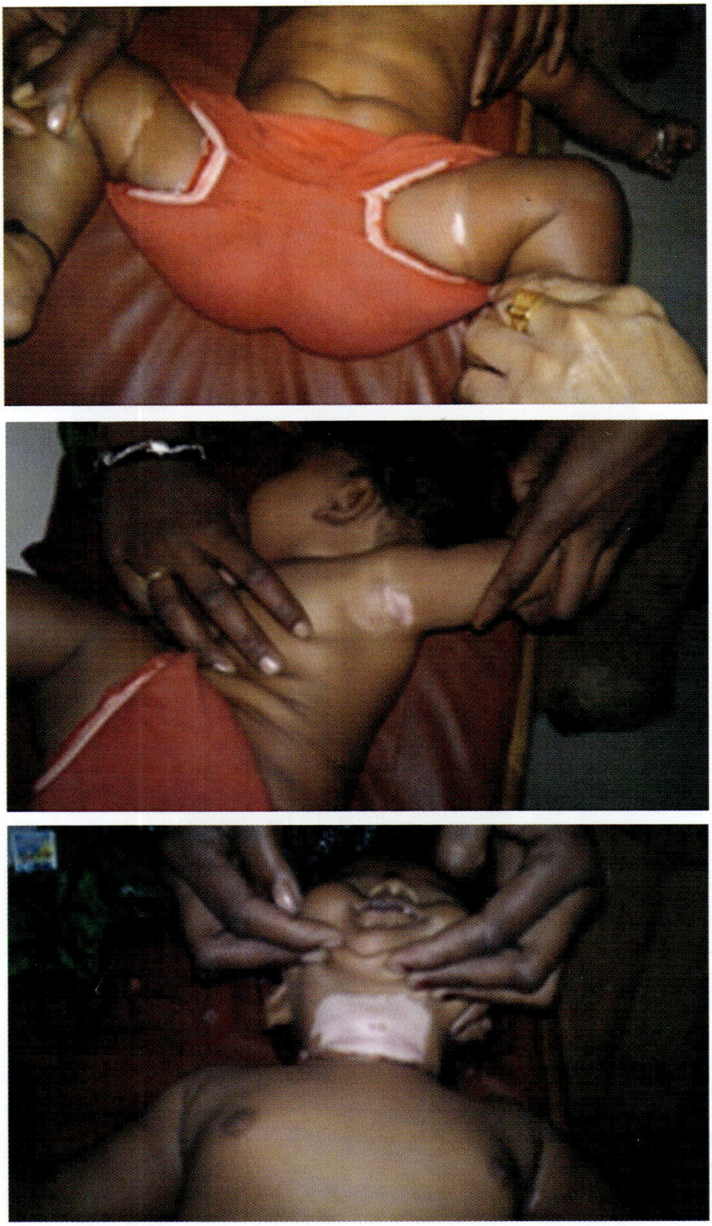

Fig. 2.6: Vitiligo lesions over flexures; thigh, axilla and neck

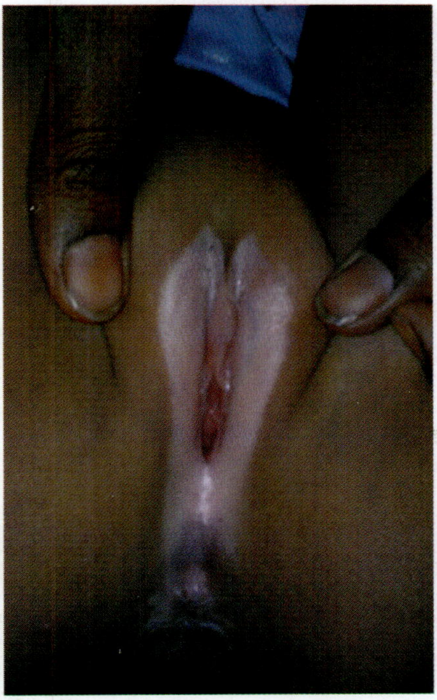

Fig. 2.7: Lesions over genitalia and perineum

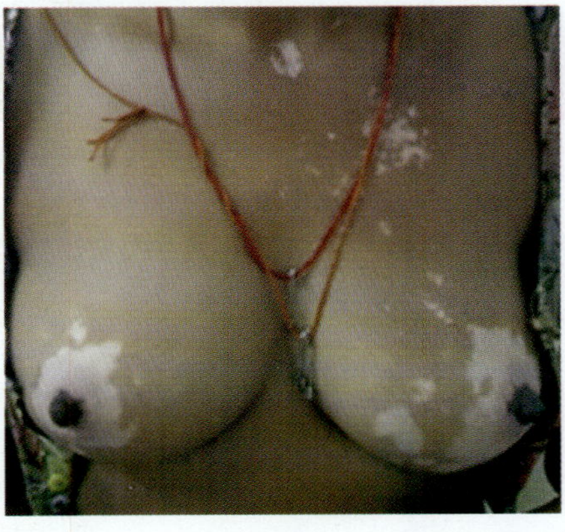

Fig. 2.8: Lesions involving both areolae. Areola is a common site for initial lesions of vitiligo

- Lesions are also distinctly more common on sites exposed to trauma (koebnerization) such as elbows, knees and fingertips (Figs. 2.4 and 2.9).

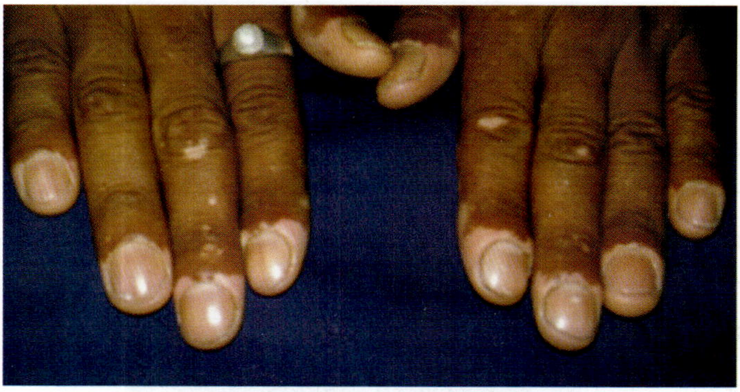

Fig. 2.9: Vitiligo affecting fingertips

- A very common site in the Indian context is the flank region due to trauma associated with tight wearing of a dhoti or saree (Figs. 2.10 and 2.11).

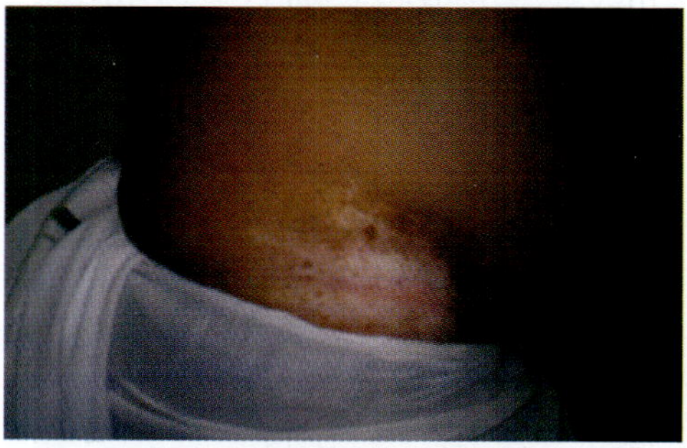

Fig. 2.10: Koebnerization in vitiligo seen over right flank due to wearing of dhoti. Common pattern seen in Indian patients

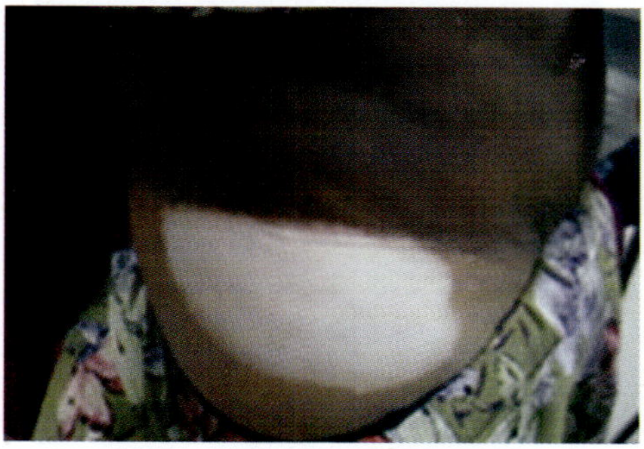

Fig. 2.11: Vitiligo lesions in a female over pressure points due to wearing a saree

- The lesions progress in size (centrifugally) and number over a period of time.
- The hair in the lesions may remain pigmented or become white (leukotrichia).
- The disease may affect one or more of skin, hair or mucous membranes.
- The lesions may demonstrate transient erythema and are prone to sunburn (Fig. 2.30).
- Some patients may also show hypopigmented lesions along with the classical depigmentation (trichrome vitiligo). Dark skinned individuals may also have perilesional hyper pigmentation following ultraviolet light exposure (quadrichrome vitiligo).
- The lesions may show repigmentation which may be spontaneous or therapy induced and may follow perifollicular (Fig. 2.4), marginal or diffuse pattern.
- The distribution of lesions forms the basis of classification of vitiligo.

CLASSIFICATION OF VITILIGO

There has been considerable confusion regarding the nomenclature and classification of vitiligo among experts across the world. The Vitiligo Global Issues Consensus Conference (VGICC) was held in 2012 to address this problem. It adopted the following definitions and classification of vitiligo (Table 2.1).

Table 2.1: Bordeaux VGICC classification and consensus nomenclature

Vitiligo/Non-Segmental Vitiligo	Acrofacial Mucosal (> 1 mucosal site) Generalized Universal Mixed (Associated with SV) Rare variants
Segmental Vitiligo	Uni, Bi or Pluri segmental
Undetermined/Unclassified Vitiligo	Focal vitiligo Mucosal vitiligo (one site in isolation)

Vitiligo/Non-Segmental Vitiligo (NSV)

- The terms Vitiligo/Non-Segmental Vitiligo have been suggested as umbrella terms for different clinical subtypes of vitiligo which are distinct from Segmental Vitiligo (SV).
- It includes acrofacial, generalized, mucosal (multifocal) and universal vitiligo and the cases which were previously classified as vitiligo vulgaris.
- Characterized by depigmentary macules of variable size.
- Often bilateral, with tendency towards symmetrical distribution (Fig. 2.12).

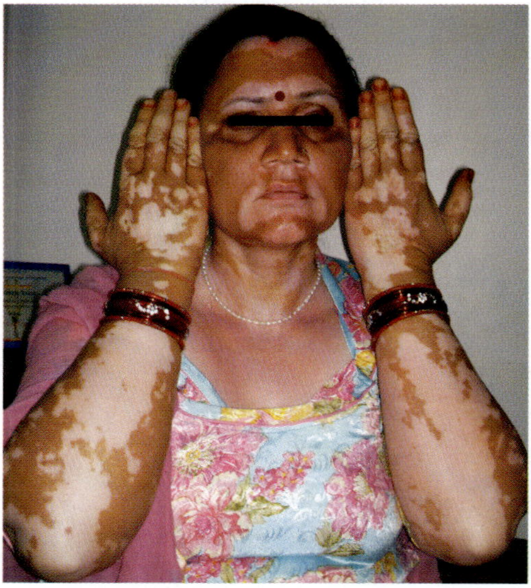

Fig. 2.12: Non-segmental vitiligo, generalized variant. Notice the characteristic symmetrical distribution

Segmental Vitiligo (SV)

- Refers to a clinically unambiguous segmental distribution of depigmented lesions (Fig. 2.13), typically associated with rapid onset and leukotrichia (Fig. 2.14).
- Clear midline demarcation (Fig. 2.14).

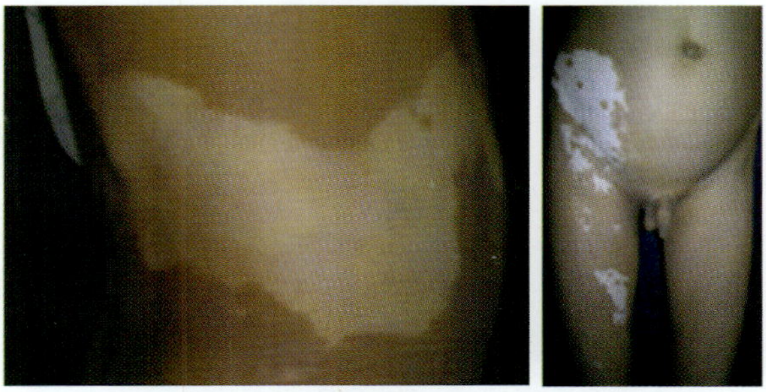

Fig. 2.13: Segmental vitiligo with dermatomal distribution

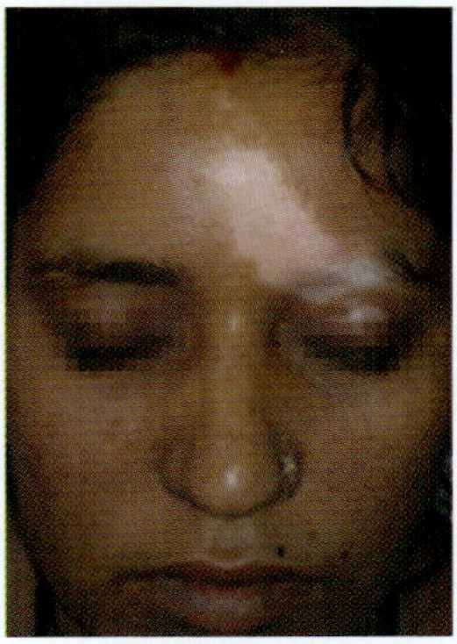

Fig. 2.14: Segmental vitiligo involving face, with leukotrichia. Also notice the clear midline demarcation

- May involve one (monosegmental), two (bisegmental) or multiple (plurisegmental) segments, distributed unilaterally or bilaterally.
- The lesions may have different patterns such as checkerboard, blaschkoid (Fig. 2.15), or phylloid (Fig. 2.16).

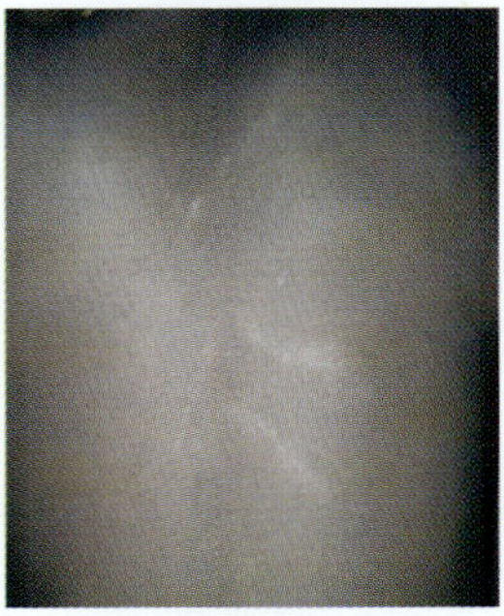

Fig. 2.15: Segmental vitiligo with blaschkoid distribution

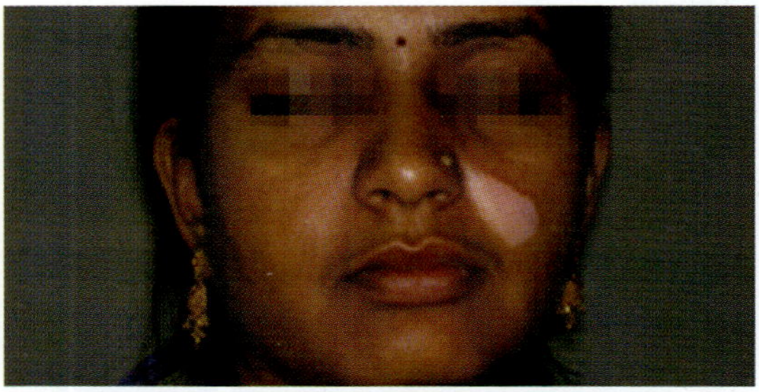

Fig. 2.16: Segmental vitiligo; phylloid variant

- The onset of disease in different segments may be simultaneous or otherwise.
- The main differentiating features of segmental and non-segmental vitiligo have been highlighted in Table 2.2.

Table 2.2: Differentiating features of segmental and non-segmental vitiligo

	Segmental vitiligo	Non-segmental vitiligo
Age of onset	Usually earlier than NSV	Usually later than SV
Progression	Rapidly progressive (over a period of 6-24 months) and then stops	Unpredictable
Distribution	Limited; Uni, Bi or Plurisegmental	Generalized, acrofacial, mucosal or universal
Hair	Upto 50% of patients demonstrate poliosis in affected areas	Usually spared, although hair depigmentation may occur with advanced disease
Association with autoimmune diseases	Less common	More common
Response to medical therapy	Poor	Better than SV
Response to surgical therapy	Melanocyte autografts typically yield good results with stable repigmentation	Response is good in traditionally responsive areas, resistant areas difficult to treat
Response to phototherapy	Helium neon laser has shown encouraging results	NB-UVB, Monoexcimer light/ laser is a first line therapy with good results

Acrofacial Vitiligo

- Also known as lip tip vitiligo.
- Characteristic involvement of distal fingers and lips (Fig. 2.17).
- Involved body sites limited to face, head, hands and feet.
- Most resistant to treatment.

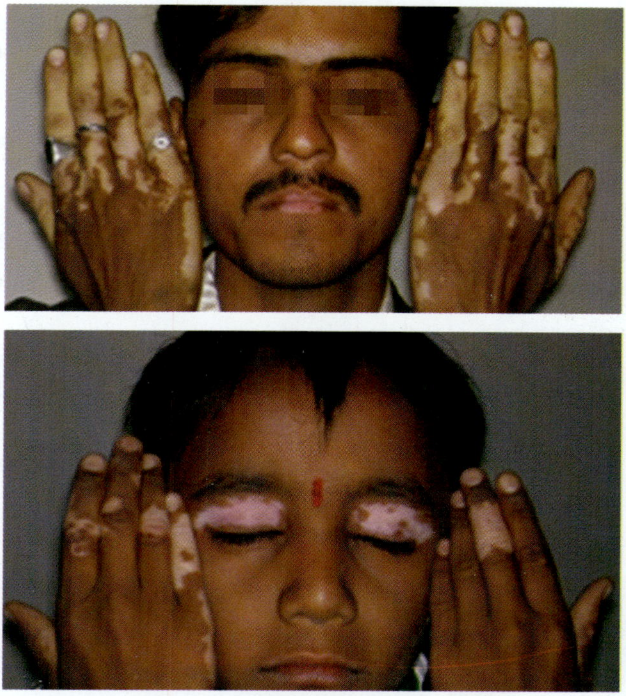

Fig. 2.17: Acrofacial vitiligo

Vitiligo Universalis

- Term used when depigmentation is almost universal (80-90% of body surface area) as seen in Fig. 2.18.
- Usually seen in adulthood when vitiligo progresses to involve whole of the body.

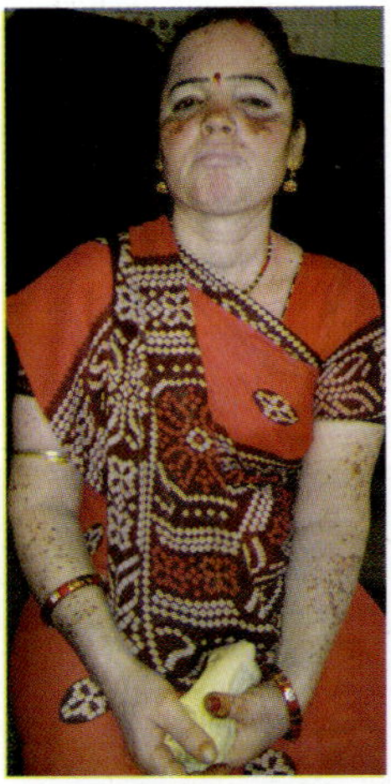

Fig. 2.18: Vitiligo universalis. Depigmenting therapy with bleaching agents is more practical in such a patient

- Hair may be completely depigmented or partially spared.
- Very difficult type of vitiligo to treat.
- It is more practical to depigment the remaining areas to achieve uniformity of skin color.

Mucosal Vitiligo

- Involvement of oral and/or genital mucosa (Figs. 2.7, 2.19 and 2.20).

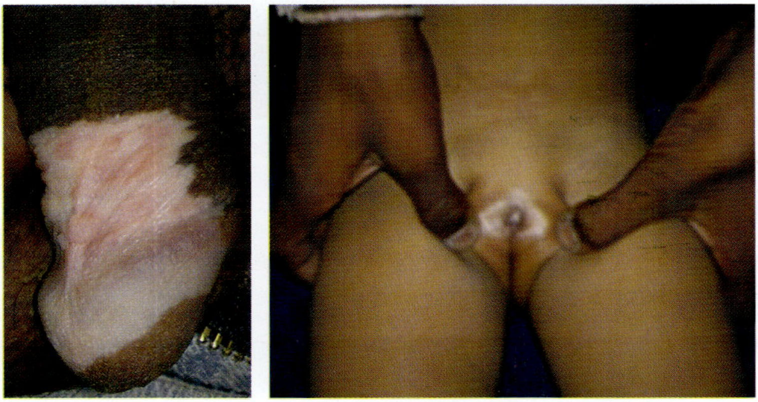

Fig. 2.19: Genital mucosal vitiligo

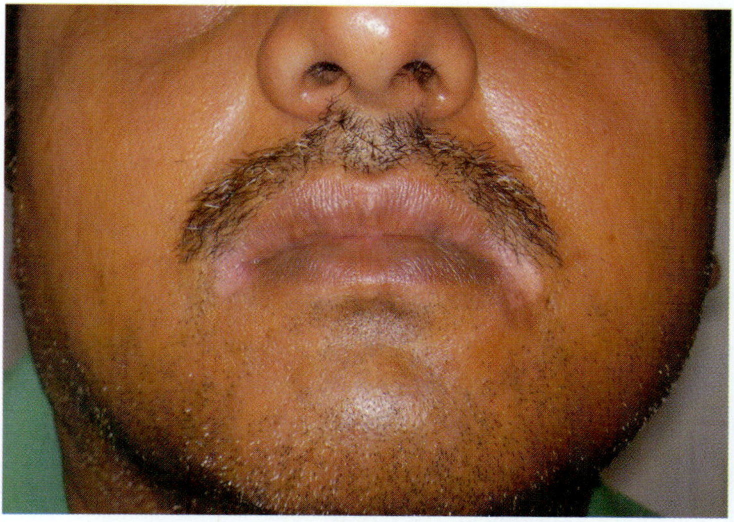

Fig. 2.20: Oral mucosal vitiligo at the angles of the mouth

- May occur with or without cutaneous lesions.
- Oral and genital mucosae are often initial site of affection in many patients.
- According to VGICC classification, if only one mucosal site is involved, without cutaneous involvement, it is categorized as unclassified/undetermined vitiligo for 2 years to allow the disease to take its natural course.
- Cases of isolated genital mucosal vitiligo must be differentiated from lichen sclerosus et atrophicus (LSA).
- Difficult to treat.

Mixed Vitiligo

- Presence of lesions of NSV and SV in the same patient.
- Usually SV precedes NSV, but not always.
- The SV lesions respond poorly to phototherapy, as compared to NSV lesions in the same patient.

Focal Vitiligo

- Diagnosis of exclusion.
- A small, acquired, isolated patch of vitiligo which:
  - Does not fit into segmental vitiligo.
  - Has not evolved into vitiligo/NSV after a period of 2 years.

Other Unclassified Forms of Vitiligo

Punctate vitiligo: Small depigmented punctiform macular lesions 1-1.5 mm in size. The lesions are sharply demarcated and may involve any part of the body.

Vitiligo minor: Refers to partially depigmented macular lesions in dark skinned individuals. They may coexist with classical vitiligo lesions, and share their pathogenesis in vitiligo.

Occupational/Contact Vitiligo

- The definition of this entity is unclear. It refers to a distinct type of depigmentation induced by contact with certain chemicals.
- However, not all persons coming in contact with these agents develop vitiligo, suggesting individual susceptibility.
- The depigmentation may be limited to the site of contact, or it may spread to other parts of the body resembling NSV.
- The culprits are usually aromatic/aliphatic derivatives of phenols/catechols.
- Such compounds may be ubiquitously present in rubber, industrial solvents, adhesives and many more products used professionally or at home.
- In the Indian context, it is commonly seen due to adhesives in bindis, rubber in purses (Fig. 2.21) and footwear.

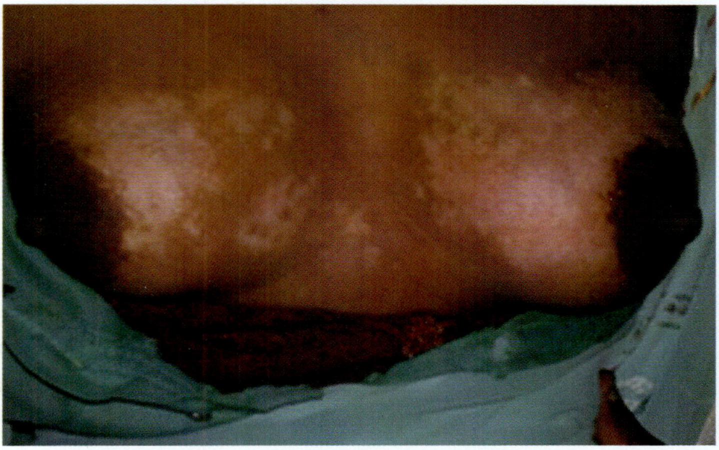

Fig. 2.21: A case of chemical leucoderma due to leather. The female had habit of keeping wallet in her blouse. Such cases are common in Indian population

HISTOPATHOLOGY

Vitiligo is a disease readily diagnosed clinically, and can be easily missed by histopathologists. Hence, it is considered a histopathologically invisible dermatosis because the changes are subtle. The main histopathological change includes the loss of melanocytes and pigmentation along the basal layer of epidermis. It is more easily demonstrated by histochemistry (Fontana-Masson and DOPA stains) and immunohistochemistry. Inflammatory infiltrate composed of lymphocytes and histiocytes, can be seen in inflammatory vitiligo and at the edge of lesions of progressive vitiligo. Other changes that can sometimes be seen are keratinocyte vacuolization, melanin incontinence and melanophages.

DIFFERENTIAL DIAGNOSES

Although many cutaneous hypopigmentary disorders may mimic vitiligo (Table 2.3), a good history and clinical examination usually makes the diagnosis of vitiligo straightforward. A typical vitiligo lesion is characteristically acquired, asymptomatic, non-scaly, normoaesthetic, chalky white depigmentation.

Table 2.3: Differential diagnoses of vitiligo

Inflammatory conditions	Neoplastic
Pityriasis alba Postinflammatory hypopigmentation Atopic dermatitis Drug (Topical or systemic) induced depigmentation	Halo nevus Amelanotic melanoma Melanoma associated leukoderma Mycosis fungoides
Infections	**Idiopathic**
Pityriasis versicolor Leprosy Post Kala azar Dermal Leishmaniasis (PKDL) Onchocerciasis Treponematoses (pinta and syphilis)	Idiopathic guttate hypomelanosis Lichen sclerosus et atrophicus Lichen striatus
Genetic syndromes	**Nevi**
Hypomelanosis of Ito Piebaldism Tuberous sclerosis Vogt-Koyanagi-Harada syndrome Waardenburg syndrome	Nevus anemicus Nevus depigmentosus/ hypopigmentosus

ASSESSMENT OF DISEASE SEVERITY IN VITILIGO

Measurement of Extent of Skin Involvement

- Wallace's Rule of Nine.
- Point counting method using transparent sheet with grid markings for area.
- Computer softwares such as Photoshop, Corel Draw etc.
- Vitiligo Area Severity Index (VASI)
  - The percentage of vitiligo involvement is calculated in terms of hand units. One hand unit (which includes the palm plus the volar surface of all digits) is approximately equivalent to 1% of the total body surface area.

– The degree of depigmentation is calculated as: 100% – complete depigmentation, no pigment is present; 90% – specks of pigment present; 75% depigmented area exceeds the pigmented area; 50% – pigmented and depigmented areas are equal; 25% – pigmented area exceeds depigmented area; and 10% – only specks of depigmentation present.

– The VASI for each body region is determined by the product of the area of vitiligo in hand units and the extent of depigmentation within each hand unit measured patch.

Total body VASI = Sum of all body sites (Hand units) × (Residual depigmentation).

Measures of Disease Activity

- *Minigrafting test:*
  – 4-6 minigrafts of 1-1.2 mm are implanted within lesions of vitiligo.
  – Area exposed to sunlight for 15 minutes daily for 6 months.
  – Pigment spread assessed after 3 months.
  – Vitiligo is considered stable if unequivocal repigmentation takes place beyond 1 mm from the border of implanted grafts.
  – Suggested as a tool for identifying patients with stable vitiligo.
- *Vitiligo Disease Activity (VIDA) score (Table 2.4).*

Table 2.4: Vitiligo disease activity score

Vitiligo activity	Duration	Score
Active	$\leq$ 6 weeks	+4
Active	6 weeks to 3 months	+3
Active	3-6 months	+2
Active	6-12 months	+1
Stable	$\geq$ 1 year	0
Stable with spontaneous repigmentation	$\geq$ 1 year	-1

- *Histopathological markers:* Inflammatory response in the form of spongiosis with microvesicle formation, lymphocytes in the epidermis and melanophages can be seen at the progressing edge of lesion.

DISEASES ASSOCIATED WITH VITILIGO

Various studies across the globe have reported associations of a number of inflammatory and autoimmune diseases with vitiligo. However, data from these studies is difficult to reconcile. Generalized NSV is more commonly associated with autoimmune diseases than segmental vitiligo. Diseases associated with vitiligo have been summarized in Table 2.5.

Table 2.5: Diseases associated with vitiligo

Diseases more commonly associated with vitiligo	Diseases less commonly associated with vitiligo
Thyroid disorders (Hashimoto's thyroiditis, Graves' disease)	Inflammatory bowel disease Multiple sclerosis
Alopecia areata	Scleroderma
Halo nevi	Sjögren's syndrome
Pernicious anemia	Myasthenia gravis
Rheumatoid arthritis	Melanoma
Systemic lupus erythematosus	Deafness
Addison's disease	Vogt Koyanagi Harada syndrome
Psoriasis	
Diabetes mellitus Type I	

MANAGEMENT OF VITILIGO

General Principles

In spite of numerous therapeutic options available for vitiligo, there is no satisfactory cure. Management in vitiligo is guided by various factors such as:

- Age.
- Type and extent of vitiligo.

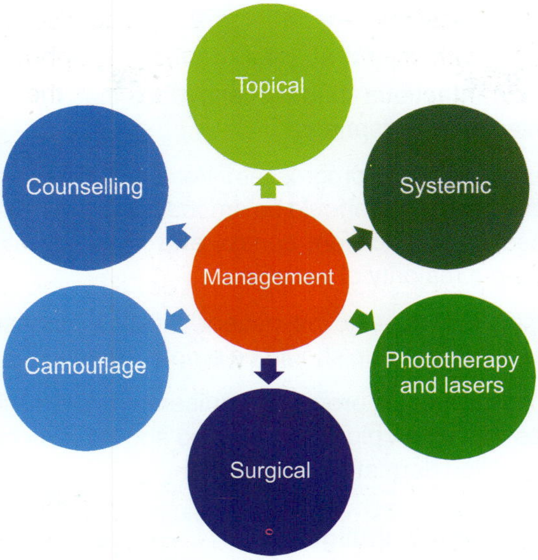

Fig. 2.22: Management of vitiligo

- Disease activity (or stability).
- Psychological impact of disease.
- Social considerations.
- Financial considerations.
- Accessibility and availability of therapeutic modalities.

Therapy in vitiligo is aimed at achieving two major goals; arresting disease progression and inducing repigmentation. To arrest disease progression, immune modulation is achieved through immunomodulators and/or phototherapy. Repigmentation can be achieved using one or more of medical, surgical or light based therapies.

Counselling

Counselling is one of the most important aspects of management of vitiligo patients and often the most neglected one. It is all the more important in Indian context because of the social stigma associated with the disease and confusion with leprosy. The following points should be emphasized:

- Vitiligo is a disease of skin color and is not related to leprosy in any manner.
- It is a non-infectious disease and does not necessarily get transmitted to the offsprings.
- Myths that the disease progresses if treated, and has no treatment, should be dispelled. It should be emphasized that if the treatment is initiated early, excellent control and repigmentation can be achieved in a majority of patients.
- The patient will have to be patient with the disease. Regular treatment and follow up should be emphasized.
- Patient should not fall prey to advertisements promising magical therapies with quick pigmentation and should seek consultation from a qualified dermatologist only.

Topical Therapy for Vitiligo

Corticosteroids

- Usually first line of treatment.
- Local immunomodulatory and anti-inflammatory effect.
- Prevent inflammatory cell mediated destruction of melanocytes and induce their repopulation.
- Stabilize progressive lesions, promote repigmentation (Fig. 2.23).
- High potency or mid potency corticosteroids used.

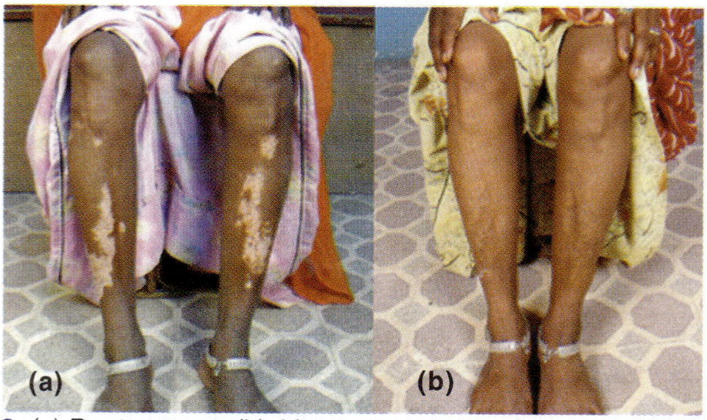

Figs. 2.23: (a) Pre-treatment (b) After 6 weeks of treatment with topical clobetasol

- Once daily application for a period extending upto 3 months is advised, both in children and adults.
- Use of potent steroids should be avoided on sensitive areas such as face and genitals.
- Suitable for limited lesions, photosensitive patients or when phototherapy cannot be used.
- Can be synergistically combined with other topical agents and phototherapy.
- Intermittent application upto a period of 6 months may be prescribed as initial or maintenance therapy to avoid local adverse effects such as epidermal atrophy, striae, steroid folliculitis and telangiectasias.
- Clobetasol propionate 0.05%, halobetasol propionate 0.05%, fluticasone propionate 0.05%, and mometasone furoate 0.1% commonly used.

Calcineurin Inhibitors

- Local immunomodulatory and anti-inflammatory effect.
- Promote melanocyte growth and migration via release of Stem Cell Factor (SCF) and Matrix Metalloproteinase 9 (MMP-9) activity.
- Results are superior on face and other sun-exposed areas (Fig. 2.24).

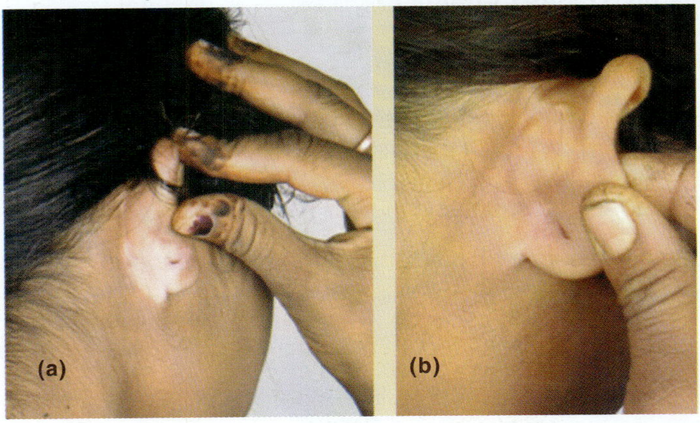

Figs. 2.24: (a) Pre-treatment (b) After 3 months of treatment with tacrolimus

- Off label use, not recommended by FDA for vitiligo.
- Can be used as a stop gap therapy in conjunction with topical corticosteroids.
- Tacrolimus (0.03% ,0.1%) and pimecrolimus (1%) are used.

Topical Vitamin D Analogues

- Melanocytes contain vitamin D receptors; their exposure to vitamin D analogues promotes tyrosinase activity and melanogenesis.
- Evidence of therapeutic efficacy not very strong.
- Cause irritation of skin.
- May be beneficial in combination with corticosteroids or phototherapy.
- Tacalcitol 4 µg/gm, calcipotriol 50 µg/gm may be used.

Placental Extract

Human placental extract has been shown to be a potent melanogen both *in vitro* and *in vivo* situations, suggesting its therapeutic potential in repigmentation of vitiligo patches.

Systemic Therapy in Vitiligo

Corticosteroids

- Systemic corticosteroids are an important component of therapy, especially in progressive vitiligo.
- Act via immunosuppression.
- Can be prescribed in conventional oral dose, depot intramuscular preparations, oral mini pulse or pulse regimes.
- There is no guideline regarding administration of oral steroids.
- Systemic adverse effects like mooning of face, weight gain, hypertension and agitation etc limit their prolonged use.

- Oral Mini Pulse (OMP) has been pioneered in India and has proven useful in arresting disease progression. It involves giving 5 mg/day of dexamethasone/betamethasone on weekends (2 consecutive days per week) for a period of extending upto 6 months.
- Not much useful in stable vitiligo.
- Can be used as initial therapy in conjunction with phototherapy for progressive vitiligo.

Immunomodulators and Biologics

Azathioprine, cyclosporine and cyclophosphamide have all been used with variable efficacies in anecdotal reports. More evidence is needed before any comment can be made on their usefulness in vitiligo. Levamisole as an immunomodulator has also been tried.

Anti TNF α agents such as etanercept and infliximab have been used in case series, but convincing evidence is lacking. Moreover, these drugs can also induce NSV.

Antioxidants

Cellular oxidative stress is considered a predisposing factor for vitiligo. A number of oral antioxidants such as extracts of *Polypodium leucotomos and Ginkgo biloba,* vitamins C and E, ubiquinone and alpha lipoic acid have been used with limited evidence of efficacy. However, they can be useful in patients undergoing phototherapy and during reactivation phase of vitiligo. Topical catalase and superoxide dismutase have also been tried.

Phototherapy in Vitiligo

Phototherapy forms an important first line therapy for vitiligo. It involves exposure of lesions to ultraviolet (UV) light, either alone or along with psoralens (photochemotherapy). It is a particularly useful therapy when topical therapies have failed, or are impractical due to widespread involvement.

Narrow Band Ultraviolet B (NB-UVB) Phototherapy

- It uses a narrow range of electromagnetic radiation of approximately 311 nm.
- It is the first line therapy for NSV, but less useful in SV.
- It helps in arresting disease activity as well as inducing repigmentation (Fig. 2.25).

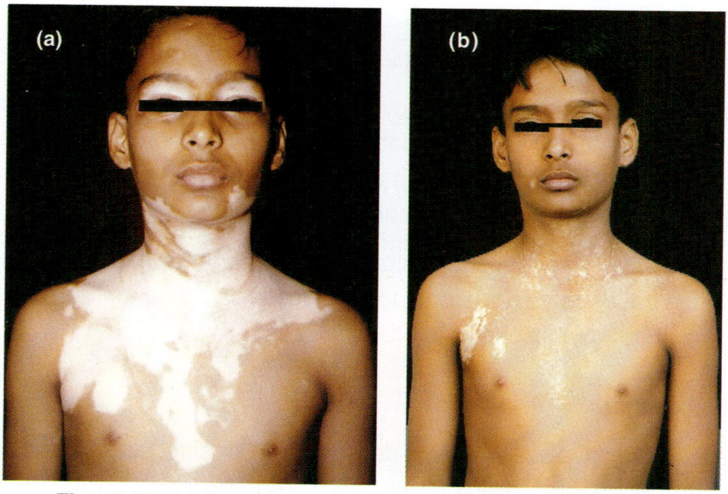

Figs. 2.25: (a) Pre-treatment (b) After 100 sessions of NB-UVB

- It possibly acts by immunosuppression, melanocyte stimulation and recruitment of melanocytes from the outer root sheath of hair follicles to repigment vitiliginous skin. Also has been shown to stimulate the release of bFGF and ET-1 from keratinocytes, which induce melanocyte proliferation.
- Its efficacy is at least equivalent or more than Psoralen + Ultraviolet A (PUVA) with fewer adverse effects. It has therefore replaced PUVA as the preferred phototherapy modality for vitiligo patients.

Method of Administration of NB-UVB

- The authors usually start treatment with initial dose of 300 mJ/cm^2, twice or thrice weekly with increments of about 10% of previous dose until a perceptible erythema appears.

- If the patient develops a burn, the treatment is halted for about a week and reinitiated from the last dose that was tolerated by the patient. Treatment is continued for about 12 months (100-150 sessions).
- It should be discontinued if no response is seen in 3 months.
- NB-UVB can be combined with topical therapies for synergistic activity; however evidence for this is scarce.
- Unlike PUVA, it can also be given safely during pregnancy and lactation.

Photochemotherapy in Vitiligo

Psoralens with Ultraviolet A (PUVA) Photochemotherapy

- Combines the use of psoralens with ultraviolet A (UVA). The source of UV light can be either sun (PUVASOL) or artificial light chambers (Fig. 2.26).

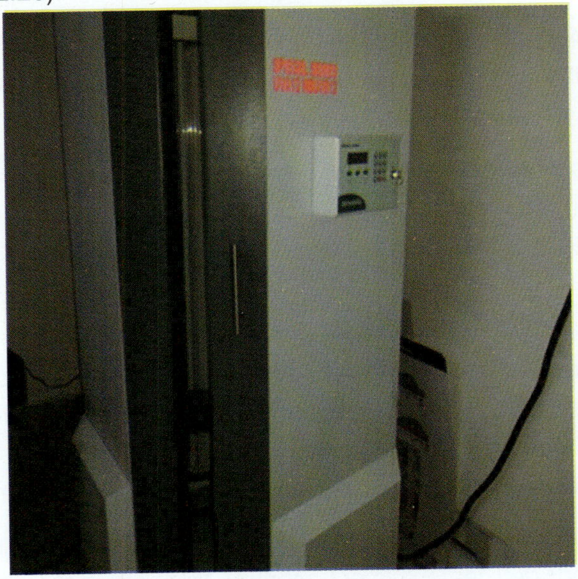

Fig. 2.26: Whole body phototherapy chamber. It is used to provide either NB-UVB or UVA

- Psoralens form monoadducts and cross linkages in DNA, which on UVA exposure, leads to various photoimmunologic effects and stimulation of melanocytes.
- 8 methoxypsoralen (Methoxsalen), a naturally occurring psoralen available in both oral and topical formulations is commonly used. However because of its high photoactivity, it is frequently associated with burns on photoexposure. Trioxsalen, a synthetic psoralen, available in oral preparation of 10 mg and 25 mg, can also be used.
- A graded photoexposure is given twice or thrice weekly for 5-10 minutes, 2 hours after oral psoralens, or for 1-2 minutes after 30 minutes of topical psoralens. When using light chambers, treatment is initiated at the dose of 4.5 - 5.5 J/cm^2. Dose increments are done by 15-20% and not more than twice a week. Final clearing dose is held as maintenance dose while frequency is decreased gradually as repigmentation occurs.
- PUVA was the first line treatment for vitiligo before the advent of NB-UVB. It is much more efficacious than broadband UV-B (BB-UVB) and almost equivalent efficacy as NB-UVB.
- Compared with NB-UVB, it has the disadvantages of requiring prolonged treatment (150-300 sessions) and an increased incidence of melanoma and non-melanoma skin cancer.

Targeted Phototherapy

- Preferred as it overcomes many of the short as well as long term complications of whole body treatment with phototherapy like reactivation of herpes, polymorphic light eruption, burning sensation, skin ageing, actinic keratosis and carcinogenicity.
- The devices used for targeted phototherapy include hand held NB-UVB devices, Excimer Laser and Monoexcimer Light (Table 2.6, Fig. 2.27).

Table 2.6: Features of excimer laser and monoexcimer light	
Excimer laser	**Monoexcimer light**
308 nm laser	308 nm light
Higher power density	Lower power density
Spot size 14-30 mm	Spot size may be upto 500 cm^2
Costlier, higher maintenance	Less costly, lower maintenance

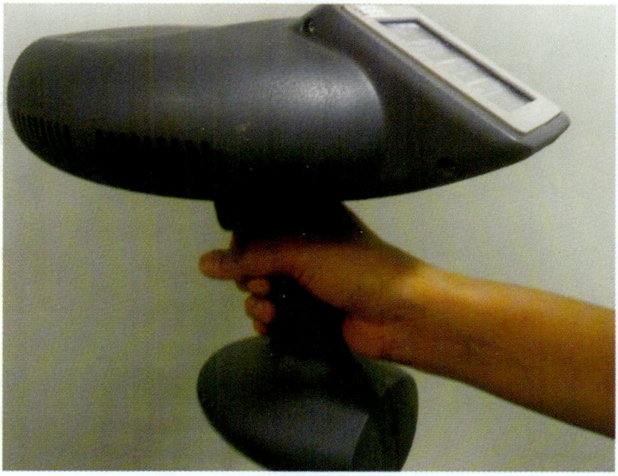

Fig. 2.27: A hand held monoexcimer light device

- Uses light exposure (either laser or incoherent light) selectively to the lesions only. This helps in reducing the total radiation exposure drastically while providing optimal therapeutic benefit. It also prevents the perilesional hyperpigmentation seen in whole body phototherapy, and thus leads to a good color match (Fig. 2.28).

Newer Treatments in Vitiligo

Basic Fibroblast Growth Factor (bFGF)

It has an important role in melanocyte migration, proliferation and UV induced repigmentation in vitiligo subjects.

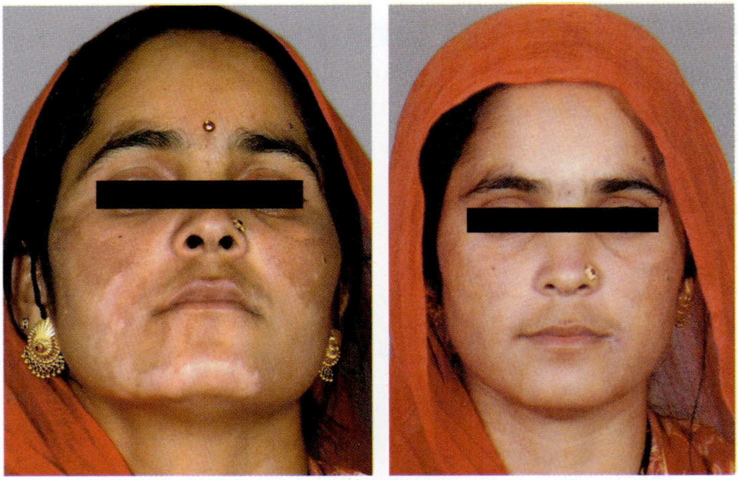

Fig. 2.28: Localized vitiligo on face responding completely to 25 sessions of MEL. Note that the patient also has melasma on face (hyperpigmented lesions)

Piperine

Has been found to stimulate cultured melanocytes. Treatment with piperine or its synthetic analogues is more useful in conjunction with phototherapy.

Prostaglandin E2 (PGE2) Analogues

Have immunomodulatory effect and play an important role in melanogenesis, stimulate melanocytes and regulate their proliferation and maturation.

Afamelanotide

Afamelanotide is an α-melanocyte stimulating hormone (MSH) agonistic analog which induces melanogenesis and skin pigmentation. Preliminary results of this therapy in vitiligo seem encouraging.

Capsaicin

High anti-apoptotic and antioxidant potential of this natural irritant has been found useful in vitiligo in experimental models.

Helium Neon Laser 632.8 nm

Helium neon lasers (632.8 nm) have been shown to have a biostimulatory effect on keratinocytes *in vitro*, thereby leading to production of basic fibroblast growth factor (bFGF) and nerve growth factor. Preliminary studies on segmental vitiligo have shown encouraging results.

Prognosis and Clinical Course

The only predictability about vitiligo is its unpredictable natural course and response to therapy. Children, disease of recent onset/short duration, lesions on face, neck and hairy regions generally respond favorably (Table 2.7).

Table 2.7: Prognostic factors for medical therapy in vitiligo

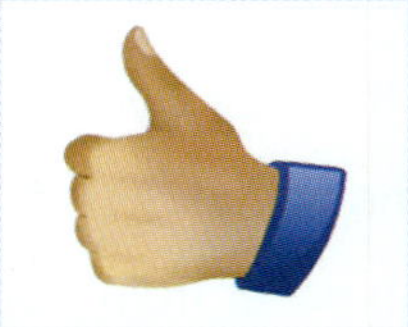	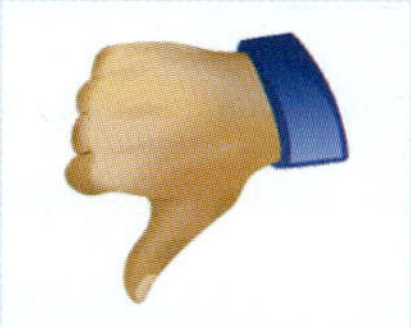
Recent onset Lesions over face, neck and trunk Younger patients Darker skin types Hairy regions Pigmented hair present within lesions	Long standing lesions Lesions over mucosa, nipples and areolae, non hairy regions, acral areas, bony prominences such as elbows, knees and ankles Segmental vitiligo Leukotrichia

Surgical Therapy

Surgical therapy is an important aspect of treatment in patches refractory to medical treatment and phototherapy. To ensure good results from surgical treatment, it is imperative that patient selection is proper, keeping the following points in mind:

- Every patient of vitiligo should undergo medical treatment and/or phototherapy first. It is only after these options have failed that patients should be considered for surgery in the residual patches.

- All types of vitiligo like SV, NSV, mucosal, acrofacial etc. can be taken up for surgery. However, it is considered more useful in SV patients because of lack of response with medical therapy.
- The disease should be stable in all patients taken up for vitiligo surgery.

Stability in Vitiligo

There is considerable confusion among experts on the definition of stable vitiligo. Various authors have suggested different periods of inactivity of vitiligo (ranging from 6 weeks to 3 years) as criteria for stability. This is further complicated by the fact that in many patients, different lesions may behave differently; i.e. the same patient may have a progressive vitiligo lesion as well as a stable vitiligo lesion.

Clinical Criteria to Define Stability

i. Lack of progression of old lesions within the past 2 years.

ii. No new lesions developing within the same period.

iii. Absence of recent Koebner phenomenon either from history or experimental induction.

iv. Repigmentation of depigmented areas spontaneously or by medical treatment.

v. Positive mini-grafting test and lack of koebnerization at donor site.

VGICC recommends that overall stability is not a reliable assessment, and careful analysis of individual areas is preferable. This can be achieved by using the combined criteria of a clinical scoring system, patient self-reporting, and serial digital imaging of specific lesions over at least 12 months.

Surgical therapy in vitiligo can be of two types: Tissue grafting and cellular grafting. The various surgical procedures along with recommendation based on the site of the lesions are highlighted in Table 2.8.

Table 2.8: Relative usefulness of different surgical therapies in different body regions

	Punch grafting	Suction blister grafting	Split thickness grafting	Autologous, non-cultured keratinocyte transplantation	Autologous, cultured melanocyte transplantation
Small areas	Recommended therapy	Recommended therapy	Recommended therapy		
Large areas				Recommended therapy	Recommended therapy
Palms and soles	Recommended therapy				
Fingers and toes	Recommended therapy	Recommended therapy			
Lips	Alternative therapy	Recommended therapy			
Eyelids, Genitals, Nipples and areolae		Recommended therapy		Recommended therapy	

Tissue Grafts

In these methods, tissues from normally pigmented covered body areas are taken and transplanted on the vitiliginous skin. These have the advantages of being inexpensive and don't require sophisticated infrastructure. However, they are suitable for treating relatively small areas.

Punch Grafting

Multiple tiny punch grafts, of size 1.2-2 mm are harvested from thighs, buttocks, post-auricular areas or the medial aspect of the upper arm and inserted into the recipient sites. The melanocytes from the donor grafts spread and populate the vitiliginous area thereby inducing repigmentation.

Suction Blister Grafting

This consists of obtaining very thin skin grafts consisting of only the epidermis by physiologically splitting the skin at dermoepidermal junction using vacuum created either by a suction machine or syringes. Ten or twenty ml syringes are inverted over the donor region and air is drawn out with the help of 3 ways canula attached with a 50 ml syringe. This is then transplanted on the denuded recipient site. The melanocytes from the lower most basal layer of the graft populate the recipient area in a few days. The epidermal graft, being avascular, falls off in a week to ten days. Repigmentation is achieved from the transplanted melanocytes over the next few months (Fig. 2.29).

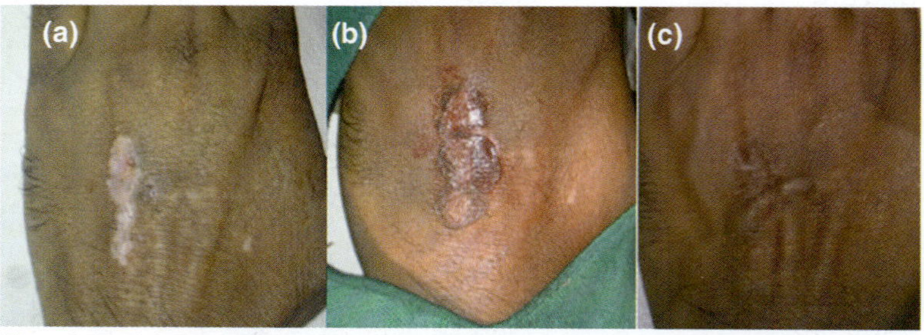

Figs. 2.29: (a) Pre-treatment (b) Suction blister graft on the denuded recipient site (c) Repigmentation seen after 3 months

Split Thickness Grafting

It involves obtaining a thin graft of 0.1-0.3 mm, including the epidermis along with the upper portion of the dermis, from donor region and grafting it onto the denuded vitiliginous skin.

Cellular Grafts

Cellular grafts include transplantation of either epidermal cells or cultured melanocytes. These are newer and most advanced surgical methods having the benefit of treating large recipient areas with relatively small donor tissue. However, these procedures require specialized training, laboratory and equipments.

Autologous, Non-cultured Keratinocyte Suspension

A split thickness skin graft of around one tenth of the size of the recipient area is harvested from the donor area. It is then trypsinized which separates the epidermal cells in a suspension. It is centrifuged to form a pellet containing melanocytes and keratinocytes. This is then transplanted on the denuded recipient area. In comparison with other surgical methods, this method has the advantage that vitiliginous skin upto 5-10 times the donor area can be treated.

Autologous, Cultured Melanocyte Transplantation

In this procedure, donor skin is obtained to form an epidermal cell suspension and collected cells are re-suspended in culture medium. Melanocytes are cultured *in vitro* for 15 to 30 days in Hu16 medium and are transplanted onto the denuded recipient area in a density of 1000-2000 melanocytes/mm^2. This method has the potential to treat unlimited areas. However, treating >30% body surface area is not recommended because of minimal chances of success.

Autologous, Cultured Epithelial Grafts

In this procedure, epidermal cells derived from donor tissue are cultivated in a medium that allows co-cultivation of melanocytes and keratinocytes. A cultured epidermal sheet is formed in a few weeks, which is attached to petrolatum gauze and applied on the denuded recipient area.

Autologous, Non-cultured, Hair Follicle Cell Suspension

In this technique, pigmented hair follicles are utilized for obtaining the epidermal cell suspension. This makes use of the richer concentration of melanocytes and stem cells in the hair follicles compared to the interfollicular epidermis.

Camouflage

- Camouflage techniques are particularly useful in patients not responding to therapy, not willing to take treatment and in whom treatment can't be given for medical reasons.
- Wide range of tanning agents, stains, dyes, tinted cover creams, compact, foundations and dyes are available.
- Semipermanent and permanent tattoos are also sometimes useful in providing camouflage. They are especially useful in mucosal lesions and in patients with darker complexions.

Depigmentation Therapy

- A practical approach in patients with extensive vitiligo/vitiligo universalis (Figs. 2.18 and 2.30).

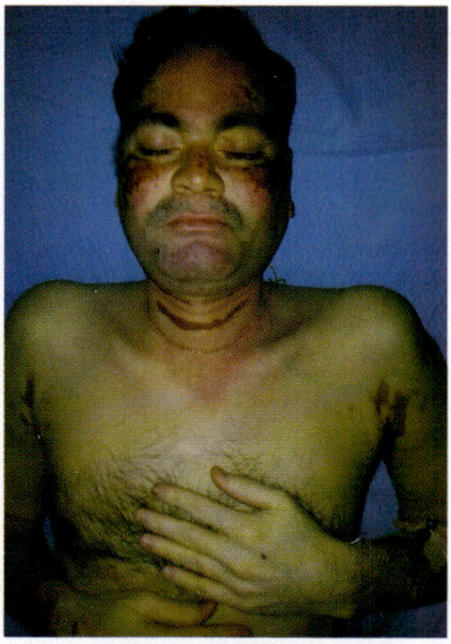

Fig. 2.30: Vitiligo universalis with a few islands of normal skin. Depigmentation therapy is a useful option in such cases. Also note the erythema seen over the photoexposed vitiliginous areas

- Monobenzyl ether of hydroquinone (MBEH), 10-20% cream applied twice daily for 5-12 months is the most commonly used agent. It enzymatically converts to quinone, which reacts with proteins and DNA of melanocytes to induce melanocyte death.
- Upto 95% of patients achieve full depigmentation, can also be used in combination with tretinoin which promotes rapid loss of pigment.
- Other agents include monomethyl ether of hydroquinone, 88% phenol, depigmenting lasers and cryotherapy, topical imatinib, imiquimod and diphencyprone.

Suggested Readings

1. Anstey AV; *Disorders of Skin Colour,* In: Burns T, Breathnach S, Cox N, Griffiths C, eds.; *Rook's Textbook of Dermatology,* 8th edn., West Sussex, UK: Wiley-Blackwell 2010, pp. 58.46-58.49.
2. Picardo M, Taïeb A, eds.; *Vitiligo,* New York: Springer; 2010.
3. Ezzedine K, Lim H W, Suzuki T, Katayama I, Hamzavi I, Lan CCE; *et al. Revised Classification/Nomenclature of Vitiligo and Related Issues: The Vitiligo Global Issues Consensus Conference*; Pigment Cell Melanoma Res 2012 May 25(3): pp. E1-13.
4. Alikhan A, Felsten LM, Daly M, Petronic-Rosic V; *Vitiligo: A Comprehensive Overview Part I. Introduction, Epidemiology, Quality of Life, Diagnosis, Differential Diagnosis, Associations, Histopathology, Etiology and Work-up; J Am Acad Dermatol* 2011;65: pp. 473-91.
5. Felsten LM, Alikhan A, Petronic-Rosic V; *Vitiligo: A Comprehensive Overview Part II: Treatment Options and Approach to Treatment; J Am Acad Dermatol* 2011;65: pp. 493-514.
6. Prasad D, Gupta S; *Standard Guidelines of Care for Vitiligo Surgery; Indian J Dermatol Venereol Leprol* 2008;74: pp. S37-S45.
7. Taieb A, Alomar A, Böhm M, Dell'Anna ML, De Pase A, Eleftheriadou V; *et al. Guidelines for the Management of Vitiligo: The European Dermatology Forum Consensus* 2013;68: pp. 5-19.
8. Khanna N, editor; *Illustrated Synopsis of Dermatology and Sexually Transmitted Diseases,* Delhi: Peepee Publishers and Distributors (P) Ltd 2005, pp. 117-22.
9. Lahiri K, Chatterjee M, Sarkar R, eds.; *Pigmentary Disorders, A Comprehensive Compendium,* New Delhi: Jaypee Brothers Medical Publishers (P) Ltd; 2014.

3 Hypopigmentary Disorders Other Than Vitiligo

Lalit K Gupta, Ashok K Khare, Nidheesh Agarwal, Chesta Agrawal

Chapter At A Glance

- Not all hypopigmented cutaneous lesions should be confused with vitiligo.
- Many conditions with diverse etiology may present as cutaneous hypopigmentation.
- These conditions may present since birth or acquired later in life.
- The hypopigmentation may be generalized or localized.
- Chemical leucoderma, nevus depigmentosus, Idiopathic Guttate Hypomelanosis (IGH), Hypomelanosis of Ito (HI), Progressive Macular Hypomelanosis (PMH) and post inflammatory hypopigmentation are some of the conditions that can closely mimic idiopathic vitiligo.
- History of exposure to chemicals, confetti-like macules and depigmentation following inflammation are important clues to chemical leucoderma (occupational vitiligo).
- The infective dermatoses like leprosy, pityriasis versicolor and post kala azar dermal leishmaniasis (PKDL) are common hypopigmentary conditions but can easily be differentiated from vitiligo.
- Some of these disorders may have associated ocular, auditory and systemic defects.
- The treatment of these disorders depends on the cause.
- Avoidance of sun forms an important part of treatment and prevent complications such as malignancy in cases of albinism.

INTRODUCTION

Hypopigmentary lesions on skin evoke a great deal of anxiety as patients commonly tend to perceive anything white on the skin as vitiligo. There are a large number of conditions (Table 3.1) of diverse etiologies such as genetic/nevoid, infective, chemical, nutritional, inflammatory, post-inflammatory and idiopathic that can closely mimic vitiligo and therefore clinicians need to be familiar with these in order to avoid misdiagnosis and mistreatment.

Table 3.1: Important causes of hypopigmentary skin disorders

Cause	Examples
Genetic/Nevoid **Generalized**	Albinism, Piebaldism, Waardenburg syndrome, Alezzandrini's syndrome, Albinoid syndromes*
Localized	Tuberous sclerosis complex, Hypomelanosis of Ito, Nevus depigmentosus, Darier-White disease, Focal dermal hypoplasia
Chemicals and drugs	Monobenzyl ether of hydroquinone, Hydroquinone, p-cresol, Thiuram, Topical/intralesional steroids, Azelaic acid, Benzoyl peroxide, Systemic medications–Chloroquine, Imatinib mesylate
Infective	Pityriasis (Tinea) Versicolor, Leprosy, PKDL, Secondary syphilis, Non-endemic treponematoses, Onchocerciasis
Post-inflammatory	Pityriasis alba, Sarcoidosis, Hypopigmented mycosis fungoides, Scleroderma, Lupus erythematosus, Lichen sclerosus et atrophicus
Nutritional	Kwashiorkor
Metabolic	Phenylketonuria, Histidinemia, Homocystinuria, Menkes syndrome
Miscellaneous	IGH, Halo nevus, Lichen striatus, PMH, Vogt-Koyanagi-Harada syndrome, Vagabond's leucomelanoderma

* See Table 3.4 for details.

The mechanism of hypopigmentation (Table 3.2) in most of these disorders involves defect in number or function of melanocytes, melanin synthesis, melanosome transfer or a combination of these factors. In some of the conditions, the hypopigmentation appears unrelated to melanocyte pathology (pseudohypopigmentation) as in nevus anemicus (vasoconstriction) and anemia (reduced oxyhemoglobin). Some of these disorders can be diagnosed by their characteristic patterns (Table 3.3). This section describes the most characteristic and diagnostic features of commonly seen hypopigmentary disorders.

Table 3.2: Mechanisms of hypopigmentation

Absent/damaged melanocytes	Vitiligo Piebaldism Post-inflammatory hypopigmentation Chemical leucoderma
Altered tyrosinase metabolism	Albinism Pityriasis versicolor
Reduced MSH/ACTH activity	Hypopituitarism
Abnormal vasculature	Nevus anemicus

Table 3.3: Characteristic patterns of some hypopigmentary diseases

Pattern	Condition
Raindrop appearance	Arsenicosis
Salt pepper appearance	Systemic sclerosis
Necklace of Venus	Syphilis
Ash leaf macules	Tuberous sclerosis
Leopard skin appearance	Onchocerciasis
Porcelain white depigmentation	Degos' disease, IGH

GENETIC/NEVOID HYPOPIGMENTARY DISORDERS

Oculocutaneous Albinism (OCA)

- Autosomal recessive inheritance with a prevalence of 1 in 10,000.

- Two main variants are: (a) Tyrosinase positive (less severe) and (b) Tyrosinase negative (more severe), *based on hair bulb test* **(**Plucked hair from tyrosinase-positive albinism when incubated in DOPA turn black).
- Molecular defect is absence or reduced production of melanin.
- Characterized by complete absence of melanin in skin (leucoderma), hair (poliosis) and eyes since birth (Fig. 3.1). Some pigment in skin and hair may develop with time in tyrosinase-positive patients. Depigmentation since birth, eye changes and lack of response to treatment help to differentiate OCA from vitiligo.

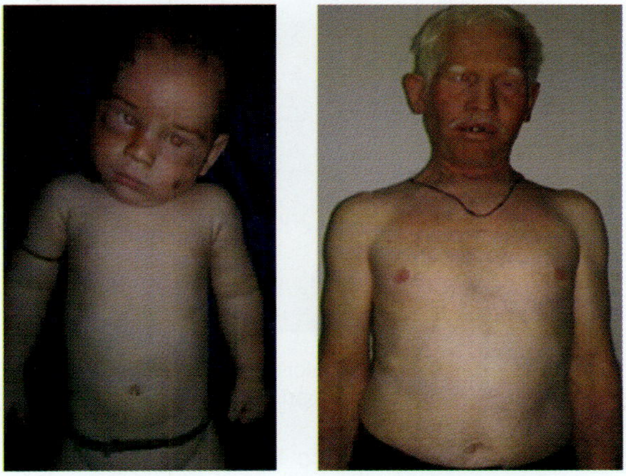

Fig. 3.1: Albinism in a child and an adult. Note the red glow in the eyes

- Eye involvement almost always present.
- Ocular complications include photophobia, poor vision and nystagmus.
- Small stature and mental retardation may be seen.
- Patients may develop UV radiation induced skin carcinomas.

Piebaldism

- Autosomal dominant.
- Melanocytes are absent in affected areas.

- Characterized by vitiligo like depigmented patches with characteristic islands of normomelanotic or hypermelanotic macules within area of depigmentation (Fig. 3.2), present since birth. The lesions remain relatively fixed throughout life.

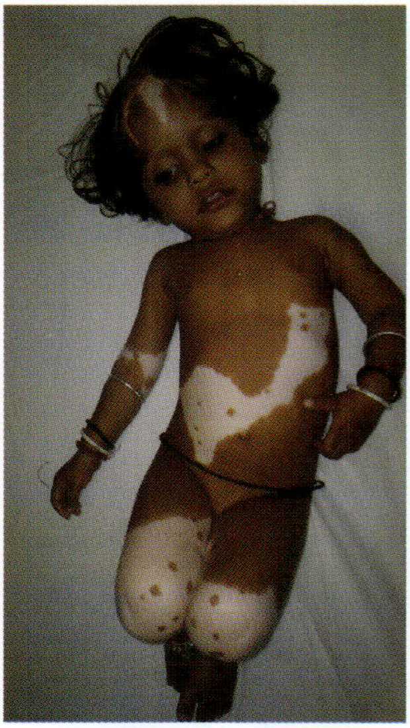

Fig. 3.2: Characteristic lesions of piebaldism in a child. Note the white forelock, pigmentary islands in the lesions and sparing of the acral parts

- The distribution of amelanotic lesions is typically median or paramedian, symmetrical, involving face, anterior chest and abdomen, mid-arms to mid-forearms and mid-thigh to mid-calves. Posterior midline, shoulders, hands, feet and periorificial areas are typically spared.
- Median or para-median white forelock (Fig. 3.3) on forehead is characteristic, seen in about 90% cases and in 10-20% may be the only presentation of piebaldism.
- Characteristic distribution with sparing of acral parts and posterior midline, presence of hyperpigmented areas in the amelanotic lesions and white forelock are features that help to differentiate piebaldism from vitiligo.

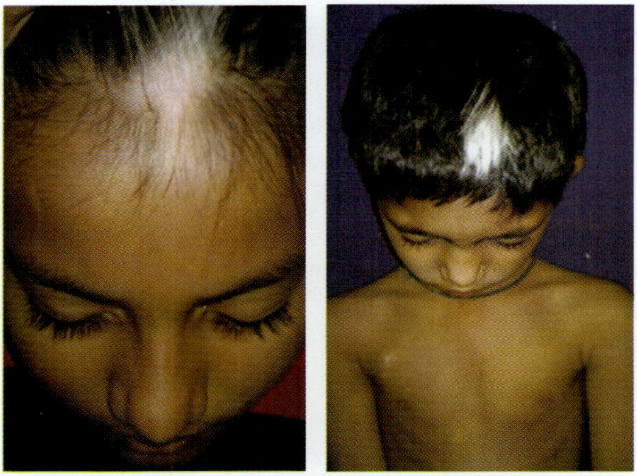

Fig. 3.3: Characteristic white forelock in patients with piebaldism

Waardenburg Syndrome

- Autosomal dominant or recessive disorder, presumed to be due to defect in the development of neural crest.
- Characterized by piebaldism like achromia of the hair or skin or both, congenital sensorineural deafness, partial or total heterochromia irides, medial eyebrow hyperplasia (synophrys), a broad nasal root and dystopia canthorum (lateral displacement of inner canthi of eyes).

Albinoid Syndromes

The entities included under this head have features resembling albinism. Many of these conditions, in addition, have associated systemic manifestations. These conditions are characterized by defective melanosome biogenesis/transport. The features of various albinoid syndromes have been summarized in Table 3.4.

Tuberous Sclerosis Complex (TSC)

- Autosomal dominant inheritance.
- Triad of facial angiofibromas (known by misnomer "adenoma sebaceum"), seizures and mental retardation.

Table 3.4: Albinoid syndromes

Syndrome	Cutaneous findings	Associated features
Hermansky-Pudlak Syndrome (HPS)	Pigmentary dilution of the skin, hair and eyes	Nystagmus, reduced visual acuity,bleeding tendency, pulmonary fibrosis, granulomatous colitis, renal failure
Chediak-Higashi Syndrome (CHS)	Partial OCA with blonde hair	Photophobia, nystagmus, bleeding diathesis, progressive neurologic dysfunction, severe immunodeficiency
Griscelli Syndrome	Pigmentary dilution of skin	Neurologic impairment, immune abnormalities, frequent infections
Prader-Willi Syndrome	Pigment dilution of skin and eyes	Neonatal hypotonia, hyperphagia and obesity, behavioral abnormalities
Phenylketonuria	Hypopigmentation of skin and hair	Seizures, microcephaly, learning disabilities, musty odor
Histidinemia	Light hair and eyes, generalized pale skin	Mental retardation, speech disturbances
Homocystinuria	Pigment dilution of skin, hair and eyes	Acrocyanosis, Marfan's like habitus, generalized osteoporosis, thrombosis, mental retardation
CROSS Syndrome	Diffuse pigmentary dilution, silvery hair	Ocular anomalies, neurologic abnormalities (psychomotor retardation, spasticity and athetoid movements)
Menke's Kinky Hair Syndrome	Hypopigmentation of skin, pili torti, trichorrhexis nodosa, broken eyebrows and eyelashes	Cutis marmorata, musculoskeletal symptoms, progressive neurological deterioration

- Hypomelanotic macules known as *Ash leaf macules* (Fig. 3.4) are often the first manifestation of disease and may be evident at birth. Trunk is the most common site. Hypopigmentation is due to poor melanization of melanosomes.

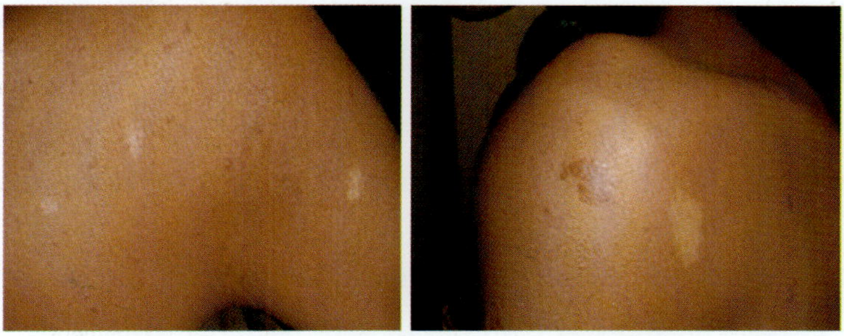

Fig. 3.4: Ash leaf macules in a patient with tuberous sclerosis

- The number of lesions varies from a few to >100 and the shape of the lesions may be polygonal, lance-ovate, "thumbprint-like" or guttate.
- The presence of three or more hypomelanotic macules, especially if lance-ovate in shape, is suggestive of TSC.

Hypomelanosis of Ito

- An example of mosaicism (clone of skin cells with decreased ability to make pigment).
- Characterized by streaks and whorls of hypo or depigmentation that occur unilaterally or bilaterally mainly on the trunk and limbs along Blaschko's lines (Fig 3.5).

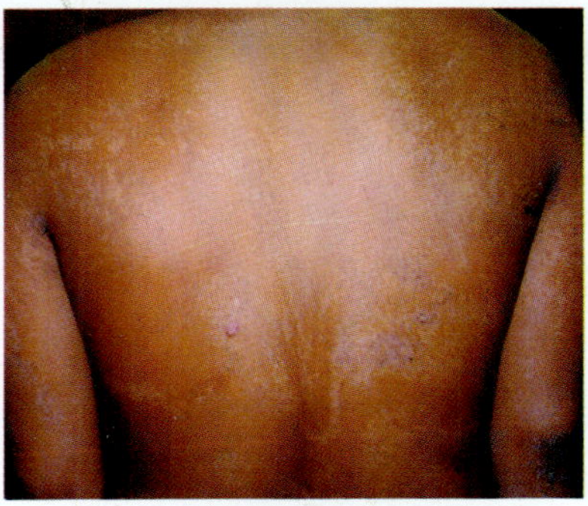

Fig. 3.5: Hypopigmented lesions with typical whorled pattern in hypomelanosis of Ito

- Present at birth or appear during early childhood.
- Abnormalities of CNS, eyes and musculoskeletal system seen in around 30%.
- Pigmentary defect may resolve with time.

Nevus Depigmentosus

- Often confused with focal vitiligo.
- Term is a misnomer as lesions are hypomelanotic rather than amelanotic.
- Thought to occur due to sporadic defect in embryonic development.
- Usually presents at birth on trunk or proximal extremities as circumscribed, irregular shaped macule(s) with feathered or serrated borders (in contrast to scalloped border in vitiligo). Lesions do not cross the midline (Fig. 3.6).

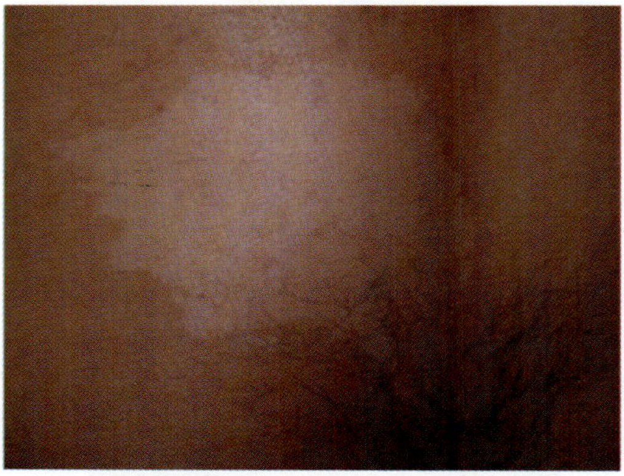

Fig. 3.6: Nevus depigmentosus. Note the serrated margins of the lesion

- Lesions remain stable, grow in proportion to the growth of the child and persist throughout life.
- Various morphological types are: solitary, segmental and systematized.
- Inapparent lesions may be visualized better under Wood's lamp.
- Needs to be differentiated from segmental vitiligo, ash leaf macule of tuberous sclerosis and hypomelanosis of Ito.

INFLAMMATORY/POST-INFLAMMATORY HYPOMELANOSIS

- Certain inflammatory conditions heal with hypopigmentation or depigmentation as a result of either direct e.g. burns and scalds or indirect damage to the melanocytes, or dysregulation/ disturbance of epidermal melanin unit. Post burn depigmentation, particularly, may cause confusion (Fig. 3.7).

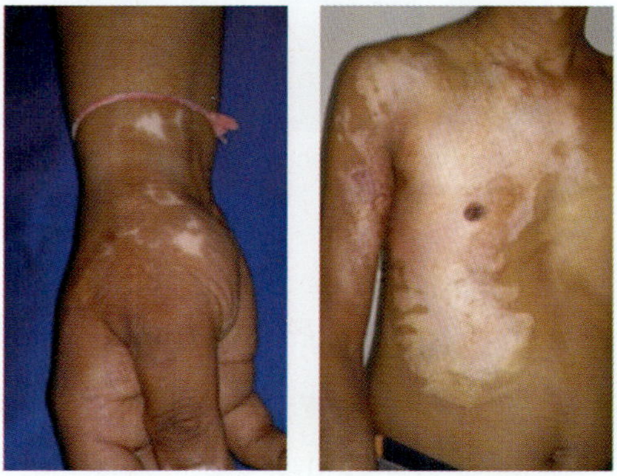

Fig. 3.7: Post burn depigmentation closely mimicking vitiligo. Note the scarring in the lesions

- Diagnosis is easy as there is a distinct history of preceding active lesions of dermatoses like psoriasis, lupus erythematosus, sarcoidosis, polymorphous light eruptions, erythema multiforme, herpes labialis, herpes zoster (Fig. 3.8) etc.

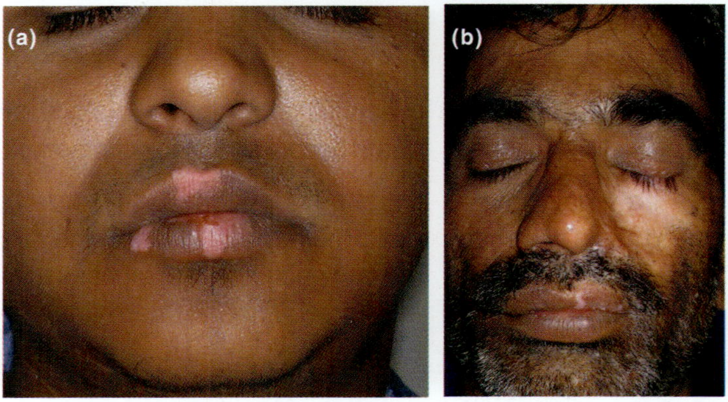

Contd.

Contd.

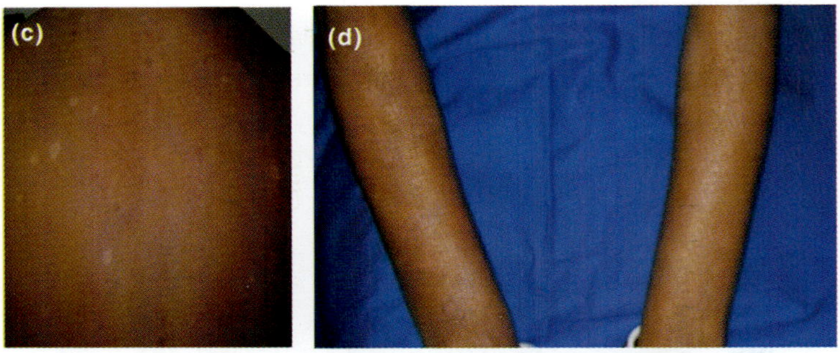

Fig. 3.8: Post-inflammatory hypopigmentation due to (a) healed herpes labialis (b) herpes zoster (c) psoriasis and (d) photodermatitis

Pityriasis Alba

- Common, self limiting hypopigmentary disorder seen in children.
- Often with a personal or family history of atopic diathesis.
- Characterized by ill-defined hypopigmentary macules with fine scaling and mild erythema at the borders (Fig. 3.9).
- Face, neck, shoulders and extensors of arm are common sites.

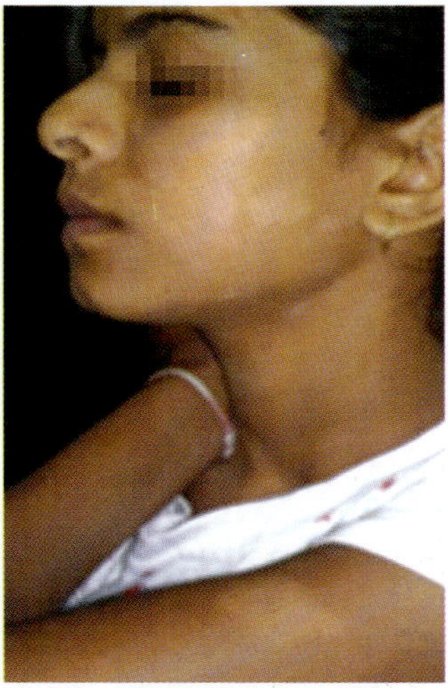

Fig. 3.9: Pityriasis alba on face. The lesions are hypopigmented (not depigmented) and have fine scaling

Scleroderma

- Vitiligo-like depigmentation with follicular repigmentation in both sclerotic and non-sclerotic skin giving a typical salt and pepper appearance (Fig. 3.10).

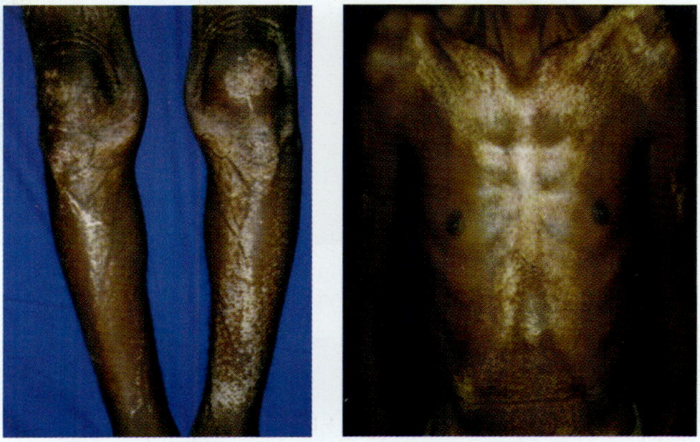

Fig. 3.10: Characteristic salt and pepper depigmentation in scleroderma. The skin is bound down to deeper structures and difficult to pinch

- Generalized hyperpigmentation, hard and bound down skin, typical facies, Raynaud's phenomenon, joint and other systemic features differentiate it from idiopathic vitiligo.

Lupus Erythematosus

- The healing lesions of discoid lupus erythematosus mimic vitiligo.
- History of preceding indurated scaly plaques, predominantly on sun exposed areas, and features like atrophy, scarring, telangiectasia and hyperpigmentation surrounding the depigmentation (Fig. 3.11) provide the clue.

Lichen Sclerosus et Atrophicus

- More common in females.
- Characterized by asymptomatic, discrete, ivory white, sclerotic papules and confluent plaques with follicular plugging (Fig. 3.12) on neck and trunk.

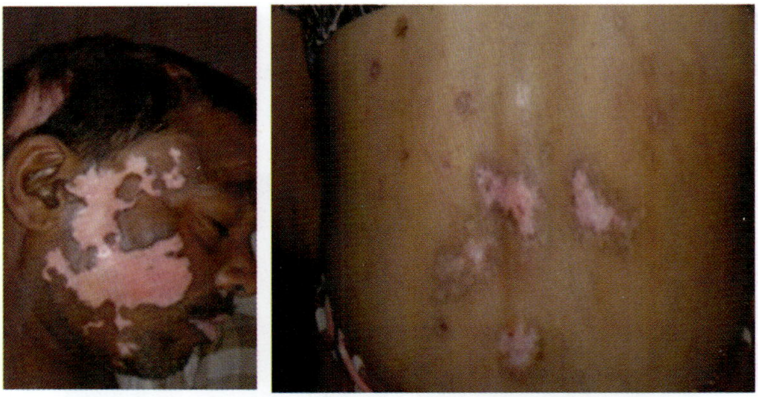

Fig. 3.11: Depigmentation with surrounding hyperpigmentation in healed lesions of lupus erythematosus. Also note the atrophic scarring in the lesions

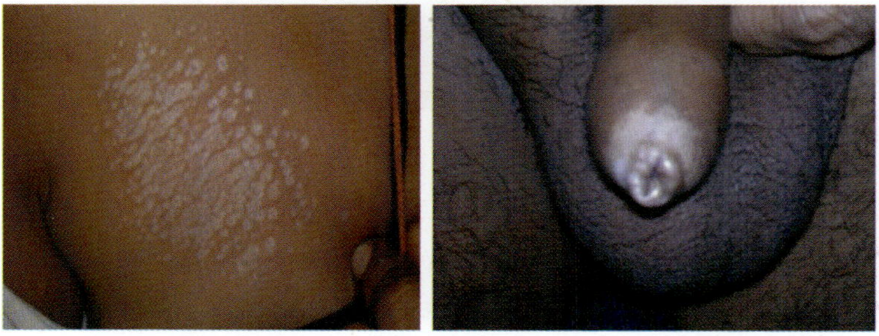

Fig. 3.12: Depigmented lesions in lichen sclerosus et atrophicus on (a) chest and (b) genitalia. Note the follicular plugging in the lesions on chest

- May be associated with genital lesions on vulva (kraurosis vulvae) and glans penis (balanitis xerotica obliterans).
- Rarely may be complicated by vulval carcinoma and urethral meatal stenosis in males.

HYPOMELANOSIS DUE TO INFECTION/INFESTATION

Hypopigmented (not depigmented) lesions are a common feature of some of the infective dermatoses due to infection/infestation like pityriasis versicolor, leprosy, PKDL and treponematoses. These diseases, however, have additional distinctive clinical and investigative clues to easily differentiate them from vitiligo.

Pityriasis (Tinea) Versicolor

- Very common superficial mycoses in young adults, caused by a lipophilic yeast, *Malassezia furfur*.
- Manifest as discrete to confluent, finely scaly, hypopigmented rather than depigmented macules, distributed symmetrically on neck, upper trunk and shoulder (Fig. 3.13).

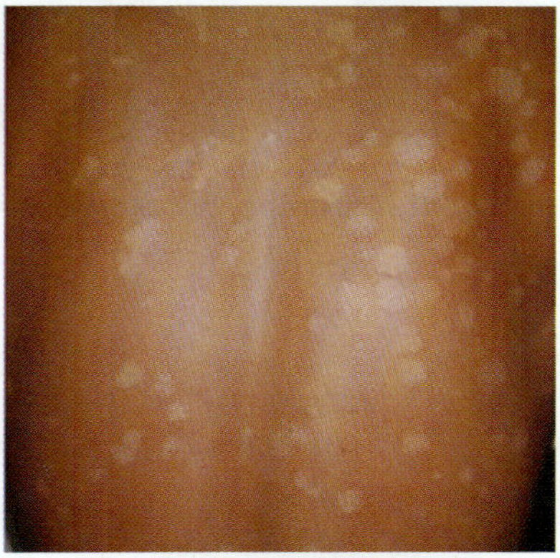

Fig. 3.13: Hypopigmented macules of pityriasis versicolor on back

- Usually asymptomatic or mildly itchy.
- Scraping or scratching accentuates the scales and lesions show yellow or golden fluorescence under Wood's lamp.
- Potassium hydroxide preparation of scales reveals hyphae and spores (*"banana and grapes" or "spaghetti and meat ball appearance"*) on microscopy.

Leprosy

- Caused by *Mycobacterium leprae*.
- Characterized by hypopigmented (Fig. 3.14) and not depigmented, ill-defined to well defined lesions that show variable degree of loss of sensation to pain, touch and temperature.
- May be asymmetrical as in indeterminate and tuberculoid leprosy or symmetrical as in lepromatous leprosy.
- The presence of hypoesthesia easily helps to differentiate leprosy from vitiligo.

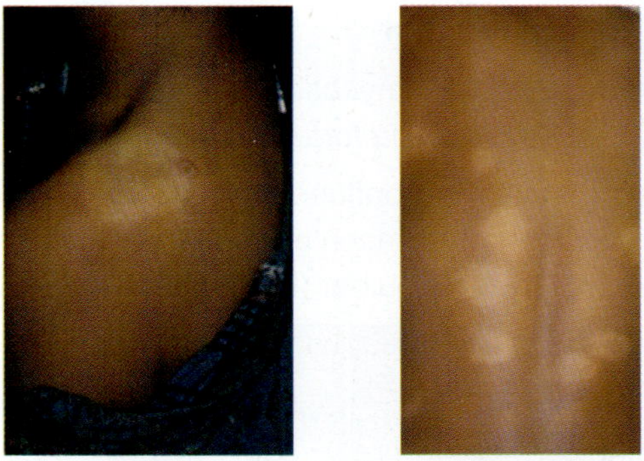

Fig. 3.14: Hypopigmented lesions in leprosy in (a) tuberculoid leprosy (b) borderline lepromatous leprosy

Post Kala Azar Dermal Leishmaniasis

- Endemic in Bihar.
- Asymptomatic, multiple, hypopigmented lesions symmetrically present on central trunk (Fig. 3.15) in association with succulent erythematous nodules on central face.

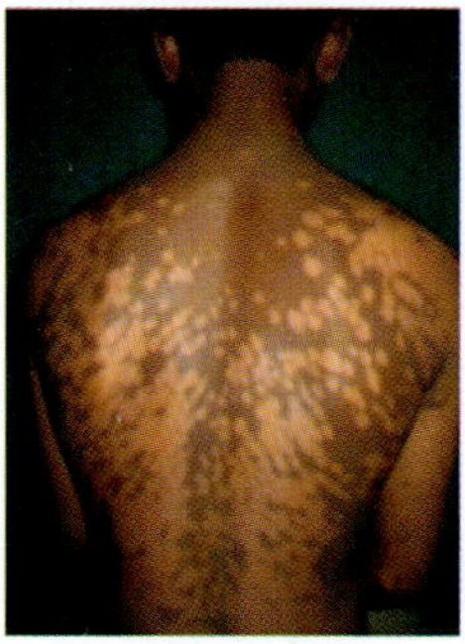

Fig. 3.15: Hypopigmented lesions of PKDL on trunk

- History of untreated or partially treated kala azar (visceral leishmaniasis) 1-5 years ago.

Secondary Syphilis

- Caused by *Treponema pallidum*.
- Leucoderma syphiliticum presents as depigmented, round to oval discrete macules around neck ("*necklace of Venus*") scattered within a larger area of hyperpigmentation on the neck.

- History of genital lesion, skin rash, supporting sexual history and positive Venereal Disease Research Laboratory (VDRL) test are helpful in distinguishing it from vitiligo.

NON-VENEREAL TREPONEMATOSES (PINTA, YAWS, BEJEL)

Pinta

- Caused by spirochete *Treponema carateum* and usually found in Central and South America.
- Depigmented lesions, surrounded by blue grey hyperpigmentation occur in late stage of disease and favor bony prominences of wrist, elbows and ankles.
- History of previous papulosquamous lesions, geographical location and positive serology for treponemal infection distinguishes pinta from vitiligo.

Onchocerciasis (River Blindness)

- A filarial disease caused by *Onchocerca volvulus*.
- Small depigmented macules occur within hyperpigmented areas on shin giving rise to *"leopard skin appearance"*.
- The pigmentary changes are preceded by itchy, lichenified, hyperpigmented papules and nodules.
- Blindness is commonly associated.

CHEMICAL LEUCODERMA

- Also known as occupational vitiligo.
- An acquired vitiligo like depigmentation which is probably underdiagnosed and is caused by exposure to chemicals which selectively destroy melanocytes. Important chemicals implicated are shown in Table 3.5.
- Besides occupational exposure in various industrial settings, several commonly used household products like sticking bindi, sindoor, footwear, watch straps (Fig. 3.16), hair dyes, alta, wallet, spectacles and hearing aids can cause chemical leucoderma. Table 3.6 provides

Table 3.5: Important industrial chemicals causing leucoderma
Phenol/Catechol derivatives
Monobenzyl ether of hydroquinone (MBH), Hydroquinone, p-tert-butyl catechol (PTBC), p-tert-butyl phenol (PTBP), p-phenylphenol, Butylated hydroxyanisole (BHA), p-cresol
Sulfhydryls
Sulfanilic acid, Cysteamine dihydrochloride, Mercaptopropylamine
Miscellaneous
Mercurials, Arsenicals, p-phenylenediamine (PPD), Chloroquine, Corticosteroids, Benzoyl peroxide

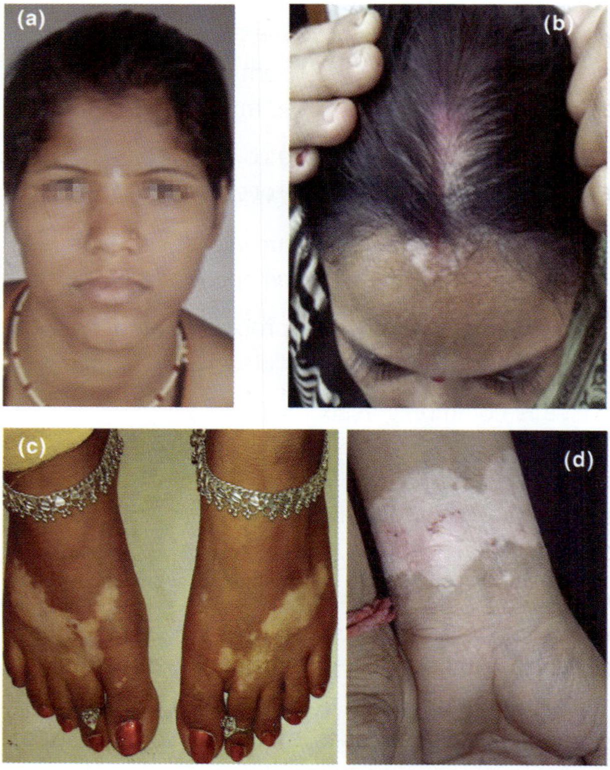

Fig. 3.16: Depigmentation due to common household objects (a) bindi, (b) sindoor (c) footwear and (d) wrist watch strap

Table 3.6: Common household causes of chemical leucoderma

Hair dye: **PPD**
Adhesive bindi, lip liner: **PTBP**
Rubber gloves, wallet, condoms, shoes, tape: **MBH**
Toothpaste: **Cinnamic**
Alta (used as feet decorative): **Azo dyes**
Artificial nails: **Methacrylate**
Rubber chappals: **Mercaptans and Thiuram**

the list of chemical leucoderma induced by commonly used household objects with their contributory chemicals.

Clinical Features of Chemical Leucoderma

- Usually develops at the site of contact with the chemical after a lag period of few weeks to few months which is period taken for shedding of reservoir of preformed melanin by epidermis.
- May later spread to the distant sites by the transfer of the chemical by hands to other parts of the body or absorption through inhalation or ingestion.
- Depigmentation often begins as small confetti-like round to oval grouped macules which coalesce gradually to form large macules with perifollicular sparing.
- Depigmentation usually characterized by a preceding inflammation of the affected skin.
- Cause can be elicited by patch test which should be read at 2 days, 1 week and for pigment loss after 4-6 weeks or, in some cases after 4-6 months.
- May be associated with some degree of spontaneous repigmentation after the contact with suspected chemical is avoided or at times depigmentation tends to be permanent.

DRUG INDUCED HYPOMELANOSIS

- Sometimes hypopigmentation follows application of potent topical steroids. Such hypopigmentation usually reverses on stopping their use.

- Intralesional or intra-articular triamcinolone acetonide injections also produce an irregular, stellate, angulated or linear hypopigmentation (Fig. 3.17) that sometimes follows the lymphatics as a streak. The depigmentation develops several weeks to months after the injection. Repeated injection with normal saline may help to disperse the drug particles and thus improve the hypopigmentation.

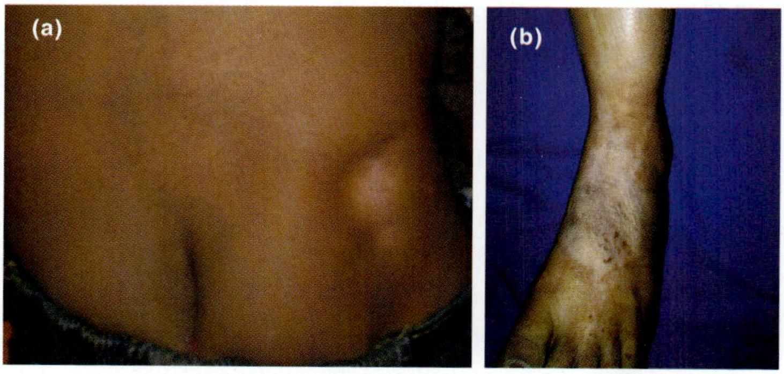

Fig. 3.17: Depigmentation from (a) intramuscular and (b) intralesional injection of triamcenolone acetonide. Note the atrophy of subcutaneous tissue on buttocks and depigmented linear streak along lymphatics on leg and foot

- The other agents that can cause hypopigmentation in skin are azelaic acid, chloroquine and imatinib mesylate.

MISCELLANEOUS CAUSES OF HYPOPIGMENTATION

Idiopathic Guttate Hypomelanosis

- Common age related degenerative condition.
- Characterized by asymptomatic, multiple, discrete, sharply defined, porcelain white macules (Fig. 3.18) mainly over extensors of forearm, shin and trunk.
- Involvement of face is rare.
- The number of lesion tends to increase with age.
- Hair within the lesions usually retain their pigment.

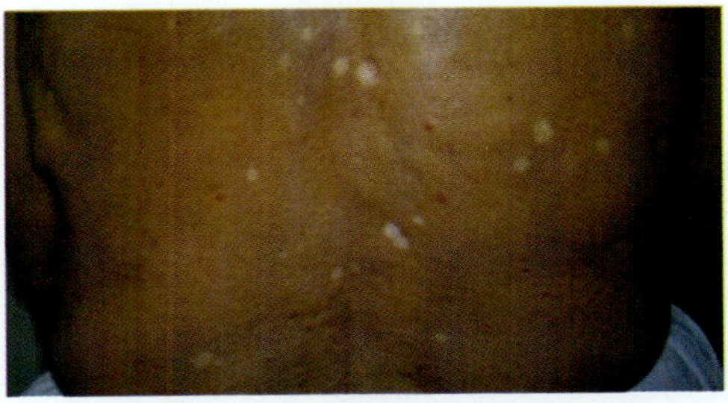

Fig. 3.18: Typical porcelain white guttate depigmented lesions on trunk in IGH

- Topical/intralesional steroids, tretinoin, cauterization with trichloroacetic acid and phenol, cryotherapy and dermabrasion may result in successful repigmentation.

Halo Nevus (Leucoderma Centrifugum Acquisitum)

- Manifests as pigmented nevus surrounded by a ring of depigmentation (Fig. 3.19).

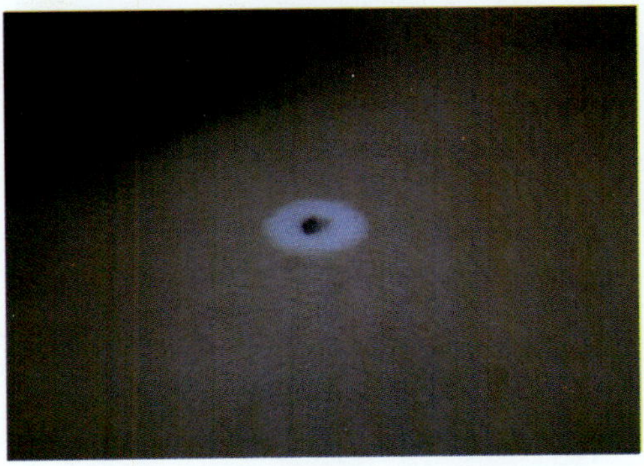

Fig. 3.19: Circular depigmentation surrounding a pigmented nevus typical of halo nevus

- Central nevus eventually disappears after several months to years. The lesions commonly occur on upper trunk.
- Besides melanocytic nevi, depigmentation may also develop around other benign tumors like neurofibromas, blue nevus, Spitz nevus, angiomas, skin tags, seborrheic keratoses or malignant melanoma.

- Vitiligo-like depigmentation remote from the tumors may develop or at times halo nevus may co-exist with vitiligo.

Lichen Striatus

- Self limiting, unilateral, linear inflammatory dermatosis in children, often along Blaschko's lines (Fig. 3.20).

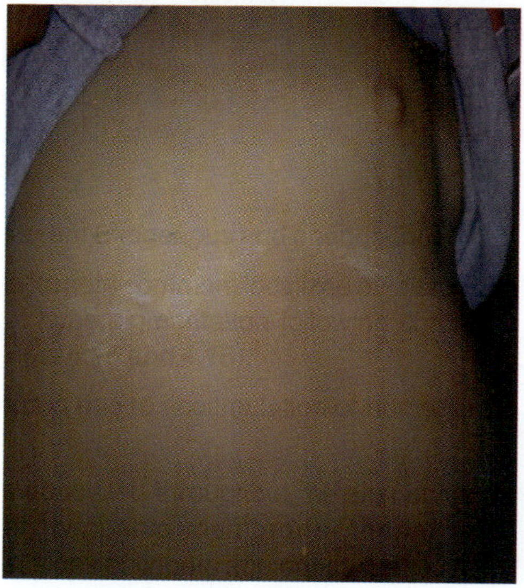

Fig. 3.20: Linear depigmentation on trunk in lichen striatus

- Often begins as asymptomatic or mildly pruritic, skin colored or lichenoid papules, arranged linearly, commonly on extremities.
- Spontaneous resolution in a few months to 1 year, however, may persist in some.

Progressive Macular Hypomelanosis

- Probably *Propionibacterium acnes* induced as the lesions favor regions with high density of sebaceous glands. Examination of lesions under a Wood's lamp shows a red follicular fluorescence.
- Frequent in young women with darkly pigmented skin. Rarely reported in elderly and spontaneously disappears after adulthood.

- Characterized by asymptomatic, ill-defined, non-scaly, hypopigmented macules and small patches mainly over lateral trunk (Fig. 3.21).

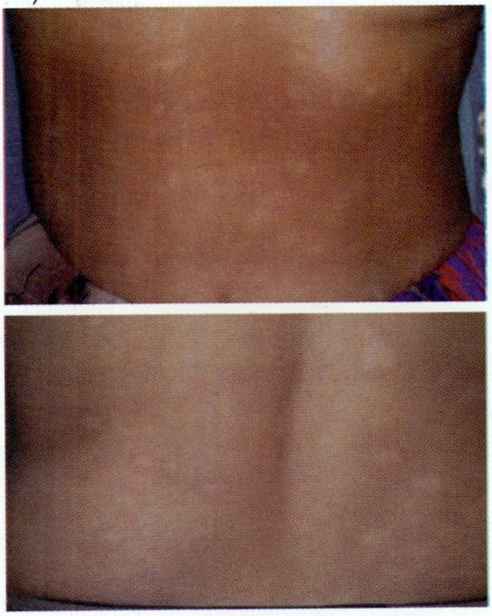

Fig. 3.21: Ill-defined macules of varying size on abdomen in patient with progressive macular hypomelanosis

- May be misdiagnosed as PKDL, leprosy, pityriasis alba and pityriasis versicolor.
- Phototherapy, both narrowband ultraviolet B (NBUVB) and PUVA either alone or in combination with antibacterial agents like topical clindamycin and 5% benzoyl peroxide may be useful.

Vogt-Koyanagi-Harada Syndrome

- Possibly post viral autoimmune disorder secondary to Epstein-Barr virus.
- Uveitis and auditory defects are followed by poliosis, vitiligo, halo nevi.
- The vitiligo has a stable course.

Vagabond's Leukomelanoderma

- Characterized by Addisonian like distribution of hyperpigmented and hypopigmented lesions in a patient with poor nutritional status and hygiene and in persons infested with *Pediculus humanus var. corporis.*

- Small macules of hypomelanosis superimposed on a background of diffuse hypermelanosis present on wrists, axillae, groin, inner thighs and posterior neck.

Suggested Readings

1. Anstey AV; *Disorders of Skin Colour,* In: Burns T, Breathnach S, Cox N, Griffiths C, eds; *Rook's Textbook of Dermatology,* 8th ed., West Sussex, UK: Wiley-Blackwell 2010, pp. 58.46-58.49.
2. Picardo M, Taïeb A, eds.; *Vitiligo,* New York: Springer; 2010.
3. Ezzedine K, Lim HW, Suzuki T, Katayama I, Hamzavi I, Lan CCE; *et al. Revised Classification/Nomenclature of Vitiligo and Related Issues: The Vitiligo Global Issues Consensus Conference,* Pigment Cell Melanoma Res 2012 May; 25(3): pp. E1-13.
4. Alikhan A, Felsten LM, Daly M, Petronic-Rosic V; *Vitiligo: A Comprehensive Overview Part I. Introduction, Epidemiology, Quality of Life, Diagnosis, Differential Diagnosis, Associations, Histopathology, Etiology and work-up; J Am Acad Dermatol* 2011;65: pp. 473-91.
5. Felsten LM, Alikhan A, Petronic-Rosic V; *Vitiligo: A Comprehensive Overview Part II: Treatment Options and Approach to Treatment; J Am Acad Dermatol* 2011;65: pp. 493-514.
6. Prasad D, Gupta S; *Standard Guidelines of Care for Vitiligo Surgery; Indian J Dermatol Venereol Leprol* 2008;74: pp. S37-S45.
7. Taieb A, Alomar A, Böhm M, Dell'Anna ML, De Pase A, Eleftheriadou V; *et al. Guidelines for the Management of Vitiligo: The European Dermatology Forum Consensus* 2013;68: pp. 5-19.
8. Khanna N, editor; *Illustrated Synopsis of Dermatology and Sexually Transmitted Diseases,* Delhi: Peepee Publishers and Distributors (P) Ltd 2005, pp. 117-22.
9. Lahiri K, Chatterjee M, Sarkar R, eds.; *Pigmentary Disorders, A Comprehensive Compendium,* New Delhi: Jaypee Brothers Medical Publishers (P) Ltd; 2014.

4 MELASMA

Manisha Balai, Nidheesh Agarwal, Lalit K Gupta, Ashok K Khare

Chapter At A Glance

- **Characterized by symmetrically distributed light to dark brown macules over sun exposed areas, usually on the face.**
- **Typically seen in females of reproductive age group.**
- **UV exposure and pregnancy/oral contraceptive pills (OCPs) are common initiating factors. Other known risk factors are genetic predisposition, hormonal factors and drugs.**
- **Often difficult to treat and has a significant negative impact on patients' quality of life.**
- **Photoprotection forms an essential aspect of management besides topical and oral therapies, chemical peels and lasers.**

INTRODUCTION

- Derived from Greek word "melas" meaning black.
- Synonyms: Chloasma, "Mask of pregnancy".
- Common acquired hyperpigmentary disorder.
- Characterized by symmetric hyperpigmented macules and patches with irregular borders on photoexposed areas.

EPIDEMIOLOGY

- More than 90% patients are women, mostly young to middle-aged (pre-menopausal).

- Melasma is rare in post-menopausal patients, even those on hormone replacement therapy (HRT).
- Prevalence varies between 1.5% and 33.3%, increases in pregnancy to around 50-70%.
- Although less common, men and children can also develop melasma (Fig. 4.1).
- Affects all racial groups, but is more common in individuals of Hispanic, Asian and African origin.
- People with dark skin (Fitzpatrick skin types IV-VI) are more frequently affected.

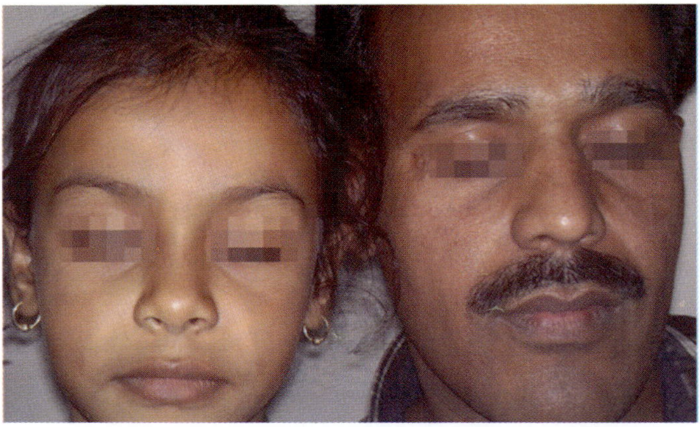

Fig. 4.1: Childhood melasma in a girl with affected father. Family history may be a risk factor for development of melasma

ETIOPATHOGENESIS

- Although the exact etiopathogenesis remains elusive, several risk factors are well-known as shown in Fig. 4.2.
- Complex interplay of genetic, environmental and hormonal factors occurs (Fig. 4.3).
- Increased melanogenesis (increased production of melanin) as well as melanocytosis (increased number of melanocytes) are responsible for the hyperpigmentation in melasma.

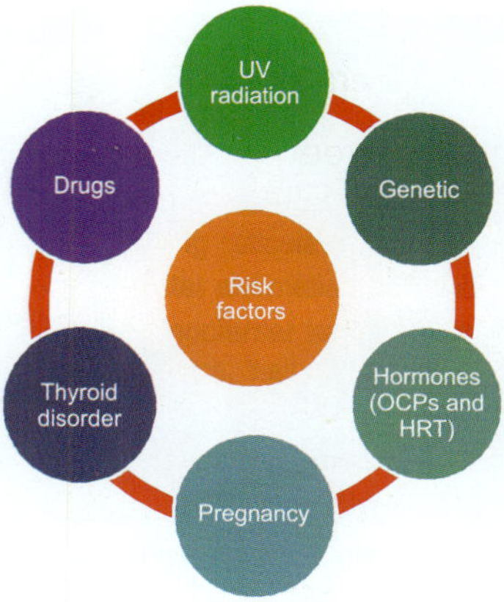

Fig. 4.2: Risk factors for the development of melasma

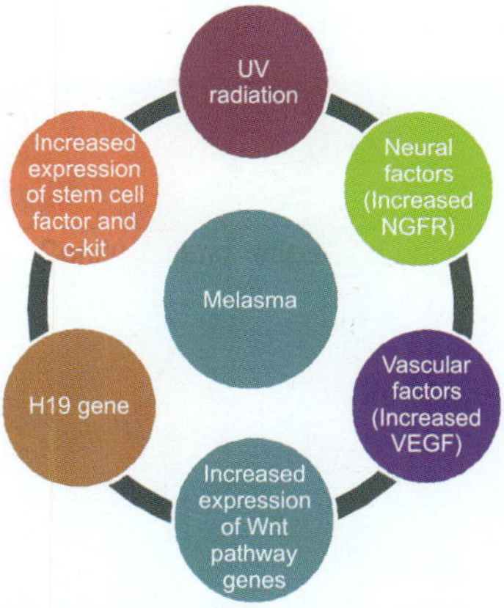

Fig. 4.3: Various pathogenetic mechanisms of melasma. A complex interplay of these factors is supposed to be responsible for causing melasma

- UV light is a commonly reported initiating or exacerbating factor for melasma because of its effects on melanocytes (proliferative, migratory and melanogenetic effects) directly and indirectly through production of various factors such as MSH, endothelin, ACTH, bFGF and prostaglandins.

CLINICAL FEATURES

- Melasma is characterized by symmetrical well defined irregular hyperpigmented patches present over face (Fig. 4.4), and less

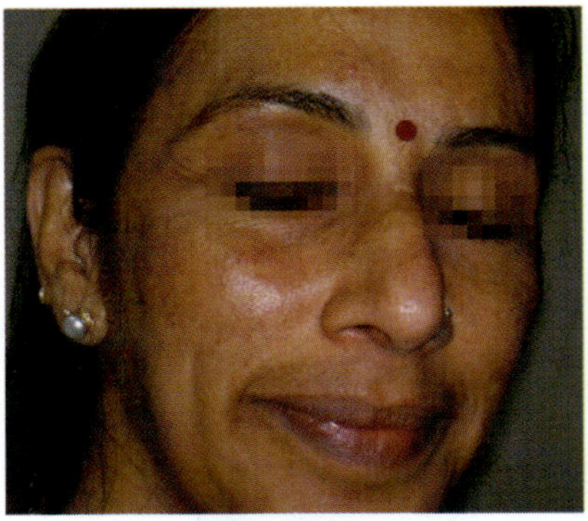

Fig. 4.4: Melasma involving the face

commonly on other sun-exposed areas such as upper chest and extensor forearms (Figs. 4.5 and 4.6).

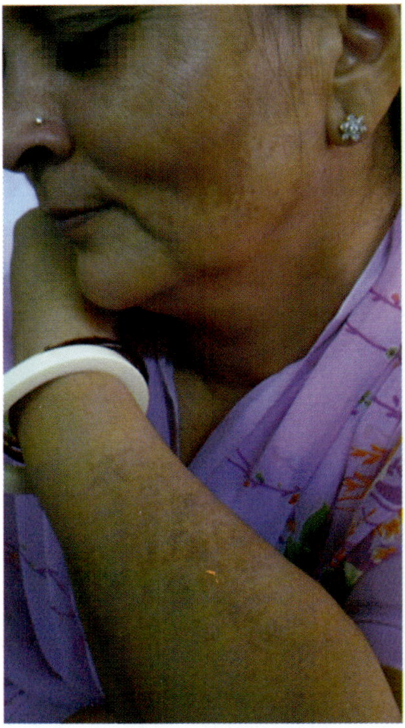

Fig. 4.5: Melasma involving face and extensor forearm

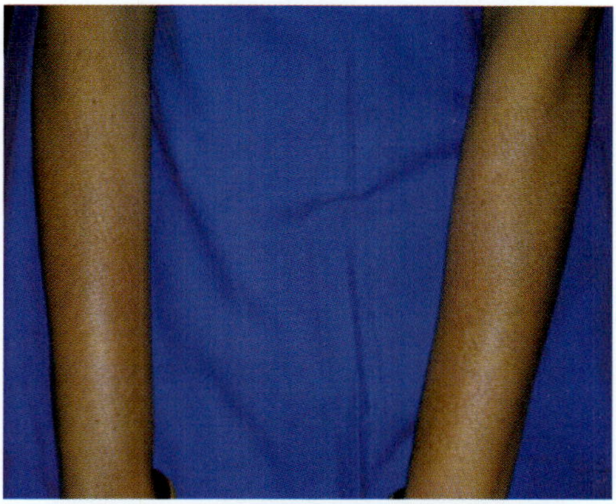

Fig. 4.6: Extrafacial melasma involving bilateral extensor forearms

- The lesions may be light brown (epidermal melasma) or dark brown/gray in color (dermal melasma).
- Such a distinction is also aided by a Wood's lamp examination which accentuates the lesions of epidermal melasma. Recently, histopathological studies have revealed that Wood's lamp examination is not a very reliable method of determining location of pigment, and that dermal melasma is more common than previously thought.

Melasma can be classified on clinical and histopathological basis as shown in Figure 4.7.

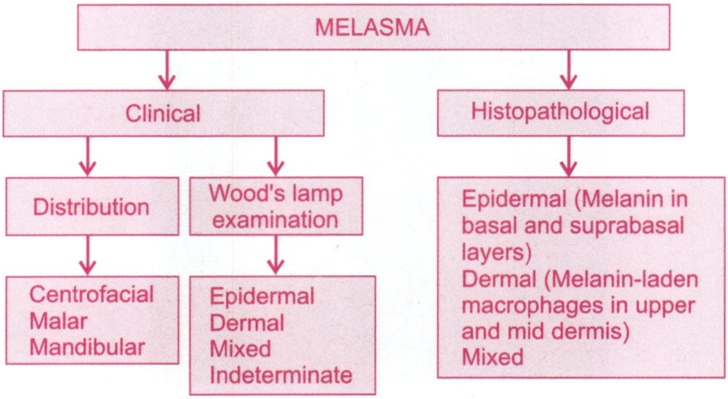

Fig. 4.7: Classification of melasma

Centrofacial melasma is the most common presentation accounting for more than half of cases, especially in women. The lesions are seen on the cheeks, lateral forehead, nose, upper lip (sparing the philtrum) and chin (Figs. 4.8 and 4.9).

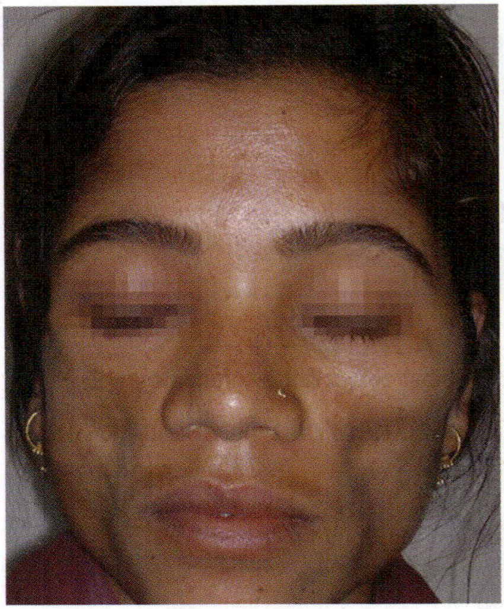

Fig. 4.8: Centrofacial melasma. Note the involvement of cheeks, forehead and upper lip, with sparing of the philtrum

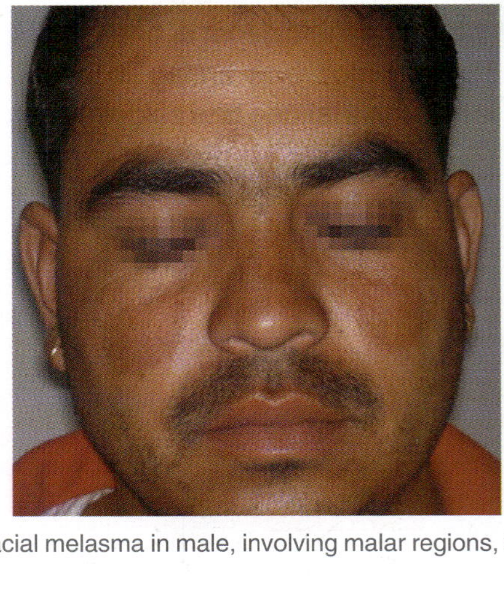

Fig. 4.9: Centrofacial melasma in male, involving malar regions, bridge of nose and eyebrows

Malar melasma is the second most common variant (21%) with lesions over cheeks and nose (Figs. 4.10 to 4.13). More common in men.

Mandibular pattern is least common of the well recognized patterns, with lesions present over the ramus of mandible.

The common initiating factors are UV exposure and pregnancy/ oral contraceptive pills (Fig. 4.13). Onset of the disease is found to be earlier in lighter skin types, and later in darker skin types. In fair skinned individuals, it frequently disappears after parturition, while it tends to persist in darker individuals.

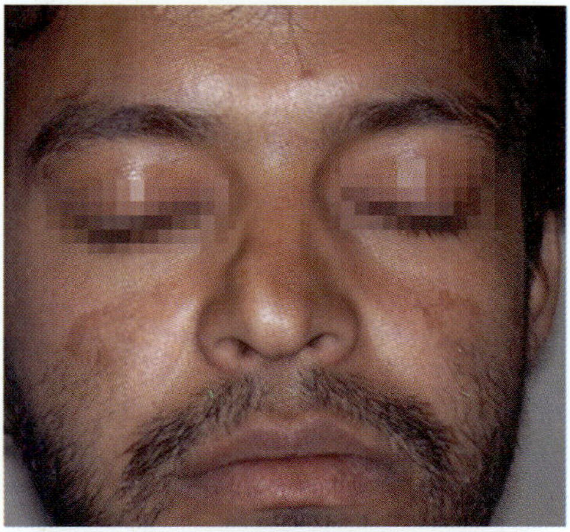

Fig. 4.10: Malar pattern of melasma in male

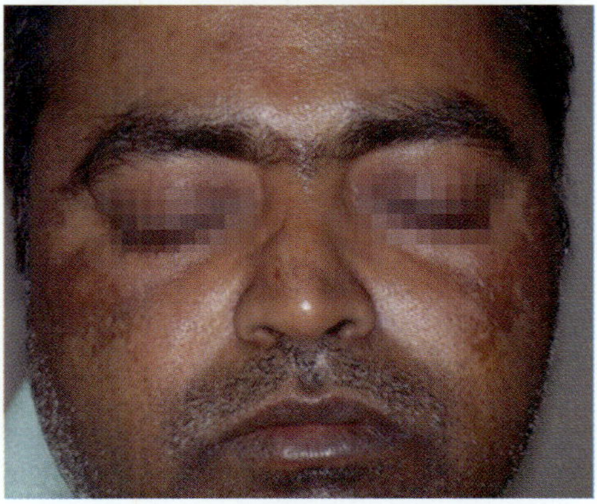

Fig. 4.11: Malar pattern of melasma in male

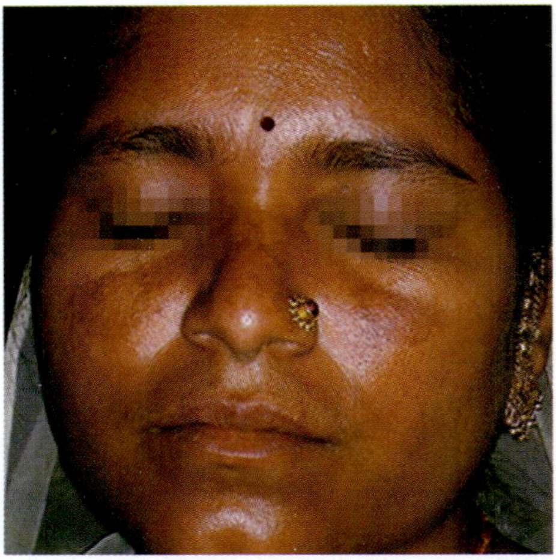

Fig. 4.12: Malar pattern of melasma in females

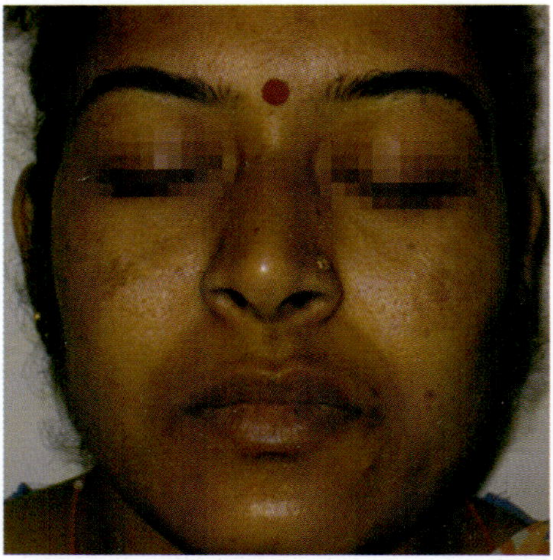

Fig. 4.13: Melasma (malar pattern) initiated by pregnancy. The patient was primigravida 2nd trimester

DIAGNOSIS

Diagnosis of melasma is primarily clinical. However, histopathology, dermoscopy and confocal microscopy may be useful for research purposes.

Histopathology

- In epidermal variant, there is presence of large, highly dendritic and biologically more active melanocytes full of pigment, along with increased melanin in the basal and suprabasal layers.
- In dermal variant, melanin laden macrophages (melanophages) are seen in papillary dermis.

Dermoscopy

- Globules of pigmented areas arranged in a reticular or net like pattern.
- Follicular sparing and sparing of acrosyringium.
- Dermal melasma shows diffuse dark brown to grayish pseudoreticular pigmentation.

Reflectance Confocal Microscopy (RCM)

- Noninvasive tool for the evaluation of the skin up to the papillary dermis.
- This technique can provide real-time images with resolution matching that of histopathology.
- It offers an innovative way of classifying melasma by pigment changes and helps in monitoring response to therapy.

ASSESSMENT OF SEVERITY OF MELASMA

MASI (Melasma Area Severity Index) Score

It is the most commonly used scoring system. Face is divided into 4 areas; forehead, left malar area, right malar area (30% each) and chin (10%).

MASI = Forehead 0.3 (D+H) A + Right malar 0.3 (D+H) A + Left malar 0.3 (D+H) A + Chin 0.1 (D+H) A

A = Area involved (No involvement: 0, <10%: 1, 10-29%: 2, 30-49%: 3, 50-69%: 4, 70-89%:5, 90-100%: 6).

D = Darkness or hyperpigmentation (0: normal skin color, 1: barely visible, 2: mild, 3: moderate, 4: severe).

H = Homogeneity (0: normal skin color, 1: slight, 2: mild, 3: marked, 4: maximum).

Total score range is 0 – 48.

Modified MASI score: Homogeneity is excluded. Total score range is 0 – 24.

DIFFERENTIAL DIAGNOSIS

Although the diagnosis of melasma is usually straightforward, a wide range of conditions may theoretically mimic melasma (Table 4.1). These disorders are distinguished from melasma based upon history (e.g. drug ingestion, previous inflammation), color, distribution pattern, histologic features and primary inflammatory lesions (if present).

Table 4.1: Differential diagnosis of melasma

Lichen planus pigmentosus	Often begins on the temples/in the preauricular area and involves the neck+/-intertriginous sites. Histologic features: Vacuolar degeneration of basal layer; variable lichenoid infiltrate.
Frictional melanosis	Lesion usually favor sites of friction such as forehead. Skin may sometimes show thickening.
Facial acanthosis nigricans	Affects temples and zygomatic areas, velvety appearance, concomitant involvement of other flexures such as neck, axillae and groins. Patients usually diabetic and/or obese.
Actinic lichen planus	Fine scale overlying violaceous lesions, perilesional halo of hypopigmentation. Histologic features: Vacuolar degeneration of basal layer, lichenoid infiltrate.
Post inflammatory hyperpigmentation	History of inflammatory phase with erythema, scale and possible pruritus or burning.
Exogenous ochronosis	History of hydroquinone application to areas of hyperpigmentation followed by progressive darkening.
Drug induced pigmentation	History of medication use.

Contd.

Contd.

	Hyperpigmentation less patterned and less irregular in outline.
Pigmented contact dermatitis	Favors sites of application of contactants, such as forehead, temples and neck. May be reticulated
Erythema dyschromicum perstans	Circular to oval, grayish blue macules, with or without an erythematous papular border. Sun-protected areas also commonly affected.
Acquired bilateral nevus of Ota-like macules (Hori's nevus)	Multiple brown-gray to brown-blue macules, primarily in the malar region; pigment-producing dermal melanocytes.

MANAGEMENT OF MELASMA

Key Features

- Treatment is challenging due to high rate of recurrence.
- Self-medication with potent steroid containing topical over the counter (OTC) medications further complicates the management.
- Broad spectrum sunscreens along with topical depigmenting agents form the mainstay of treatment.
- Chemical peeling and lasers are alternatives which may be useful in selected cases.

General Measures

- Patients should be counseled about the high recurrence rates of the disease, and warned against self-medication with steroid containing OTC medications.
- Strict photoprotection, even when indoors, forms the cornerstone of any therapeutic regimen of melasma and increases the effectiveness of other therapeutic modalities.
- This can be achieved by broad spectrum sunscreens, protective clothing (broad hats, scarves, dupattas) and umbrellas.
- If disease onset is associated with OCP/HRT use, cessation of the same may lead to spontaneous remission or improved therapeutic efficacy.

Sunscreens

- Reduce the amount of UVR reaching the skin and its direct and indirect effects on melanin production.
- A broad spectrum sunscreen covers UVA, UVB as well as the visible spectrum. Inorganic sunscreens, which act by reflecting and scattering UVR, provide broad spectrum protection but are not cosmetically elegant.
- Organic sunscreens act by absorbing UVR, but may not provide broad spectrum protection. A blend of inorganic and organic sunscreens is best.
- The ideal sunscreen is the one which satisfies all the criteria outlined in Box 4.1.
- It needs to be applied liberally to form a thick layer. The ideal amount to be applied is 2 mg/cm^2. This can be achieved by the "teaspoon rule" shown in Box 4.2.

Box 4.1: Properties of an ideal sunscreen
• Broad spectrum
• Photostable
• Cosmetically acceptable
• Water resistant
• Non-sensitizing
• Fragrance free

Box 4.2: Teaspoon rule	
3 mL or just more than half teaspoon	Each arm/face/neck
5 mL or just more than one teaspoon	Each leg/chest/back

- Sunscreens should be used even when staying indoors as diffuse light can also aggravate melasma.
- Gel-based products and sprays are better for oily and acne prone skin and people who sweat a lot, like sportspersons.

- Water in oil emulsion is a preferred option during harsh winters and for the ageing skin.

Topical Therapies

- First-line management consists of topical depigmenting therapies and photoprotection.
- Most of the therapies target tyrosinase (by different mechanisms) thereby decreasing the melanin content in newly forming epidermal layers (Table 4.2). The upper epidermal layers containing more melanin are gradually shed off. This shedding can also be facilitated by various agents such as retinoids.

Table 4.2: Mechanisms of action of various topical agents used in melasma

Mechanism of action	Compound
Inhibition of tyrosinase	Hydroquinone, Mequinol, Azelaic acid, Arbutin, Deoxyarbutin, Aloesin, Flavonoids, Licorice extract, Rucinol, N-acetyl glucosamine
Inhibition of melanosome maturation	Arbutin, Deoxyarbutin
Reducing the transfer of melanosomes from melanocytes to keratinocytes	Niacinamide, Retinoids, Soy, trypsin inhibitor
Stimulation of keratinocyte turnover	Retinoids and glycolic acid
Interaction with copper	Kojic acid, Ascorbic acid, zinc and pycnogenol
Decrease in α MSH	Beta carotene
Plasmin inhibition	Tranexamic acid

- Dermal melanin, because of being entrapped in melanophages, is difficult to remove effectively by any topical therapy. Hence responds poorly as compared to epidermal and mixed variants.

Hydroquinone (HQ)

- It is considered the gold standard of treatment for melasma.
- Used in concentrations of 2-4%.
- Efficacy is enhanced when used in combination with other agents.

- These combinations include:
  - Kligman's formula (5% HQ, 0.1% tretinoin and 0.1% dexamethasone).
  - Modified Kligman's formula (2% HQ, 0.05% tretinoin and 1% hydrocortisone acetate).
  - Pathak's formula (2% HQ and 0.05-0.1% tretinoin).
  - Westerhof's formula (4.7% N-acetylcysteine, 2% HQ and 0.1% triamcinolone acetonide).
  - Combination of microencapsulated HQ 4% with retinol 0.15% and antioxidants.
- Combination of hydroquinone with tretinoin and low to mid potency steroids such as fluocinolone and mometasone (triple combination) provides gratifying results. However, its prolonged and injudicious use can lead to adverse effects such as epidermal atrophy, hirsutism and telangiectasias (Fig. 4.14).

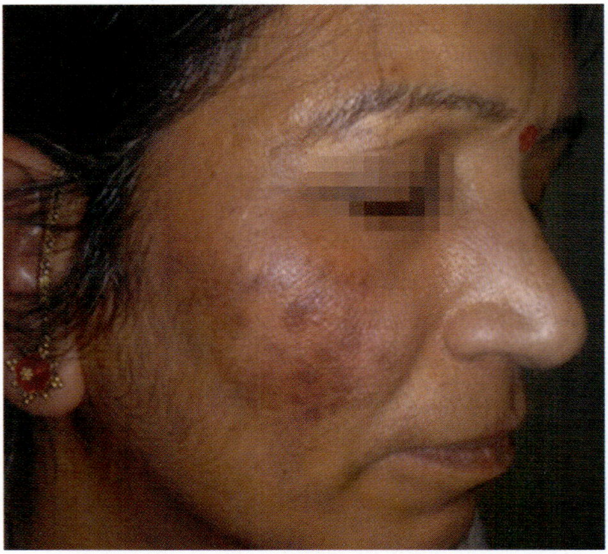

Fig. 4.14: Hirsutism, erythema and epidermal atrophy due to injudicious use of triple combination creams

- Adverse reactions are related to dose and duration of treatment, which include irritation, erythema, stinging, irritant and allergic contact dermatitis and paradoxical post-inflammatory hypermelanosis.
- Prolonged use may lead to blue-black pigmentation known as exogenous ochronosis and "confetti like" hypopigmented macules within hyperpigmented lesions (Figs. 4.15 and 4.16).

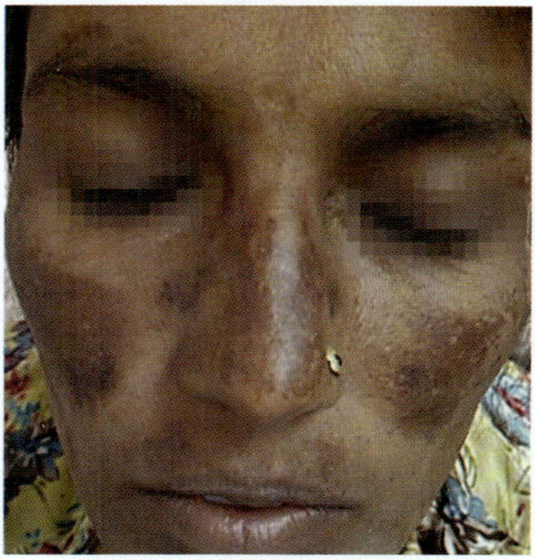

Fig. 4.15: Exogenous ochronosis

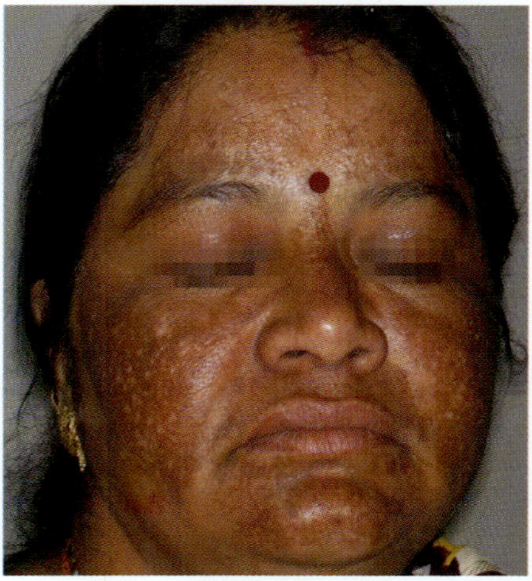

Fig. 4.16: Exogenous ochronosis and confetti like hypopigmented macules due to prolonged hydroquinone usage

Kojic Acid

- Derived from *Aspergillus*, *Acetobacter* and *Penicillium*.
- Most commonly used non-hydroquinone topical depigmenting agent.
- Used in concentrations of 1-4%.
- May cause contact dermatitis and erythema.

Arbutin and Deoxyarbutin

- Arbutin is a naturally occurring derivative of hydroquinone, found in bearberry, blueberry and cranberry plants.
- Deoxyarbutin is a more potent, synthetic derivative of arbutin.
- These agents can be used as alternatives to hydroquinone.

Azelaic Acid

- Derived from *Pityrosporum ovale.*
- Used in concentrations of 10-20%.
- May be useful in patients who do not tolerate hydroquinone and in patients having concomitant acne.

Newer and Experimental Agents

- Tranexamic acid (oral: 250 mg twice daily, topical: 5% gel).
- Pycnogenol.
- Proanthocyanidin.
- 4-n-Butyl resorcinol 0.1% cream (and other resorcinol derivatives).
- Decapeptide 12 cream (0.01%).
- Silymarin cream (0.1% and 0.2%).
- Methimazole cream (5%).

Chemical Peels

- Second-line or adjunctive treatment for melasma.

- Effective in epidermal and mixed type.
- In this procedure, a chemical agent is applied to the skin to cause a controlled destruction of a portion of the epidermis with or without dermis.
- According to depth of injury divided into superficial, medium-depth and deep peels.
- In melasma, superficial peels are most commonly used.

Glycolic Acid (GA) Peels

- Glycolic acid is an alpha hydroxy acid, commonly used in concentrations of 20-70%.
- Best used as an adjunctive treatment along with topical therapies in refractory cases.
- Side effects such as irritation are mild and may be minimized by slowly increasing the concentration.
- Darker skin types have risk of post-inflammatory hyper-pigmentation.

Trichloroacetic Acid (TCA) Peels

- Used in concentration of 10-25%.
- Mechanism of action is by epidermal protein precipitation causing necrosis.
- Low strength TCA peels are as effective as GA peels, but have higher risk of adverse effects such as burning and post-inflammatory hyperpigmentation, especially in Indian patients.

Other peels that are used in melasma include Jessner's peel (salicylic acid, lactic acid and resorcinol), tretinoin peel and Obagi blue peel. Salicylic acid peeling does not provide much benefit in melasma.

Lasers and Light Based Therapies

Lasers and light based therapies have been used in the management of melasma (Table 4.3). Theoretically, Q switched lasers (ruby,

Table 4.3: Lasers used in melasma
• Intense pulsed light (510 nm)
• Non-ablative fractional
• Ablative 2940 nm
• Q switched Alexandrite (755 nm)
• Q switched Nd: YAG (1064 nm)
• Carbon dioxide
• Copper bromide

Alexandrite and Nd:YAG), which provide laser beams of extremely short pulse duration (in nanoseconds), target melanosomes as their chromophores, which are destroyed leading to improvement in pigmentation. However, results are not satisfactory and there is a considerable chance of post-inflammatory hyperpigmentation in Indian skin types (Fig. 4.17). Fractional lasers have been approved by FDA for melasma and cause transepidermal elimination of pigment. Lasers should be used when other treatment modalities have exhausted, and with caution in Indian patients.

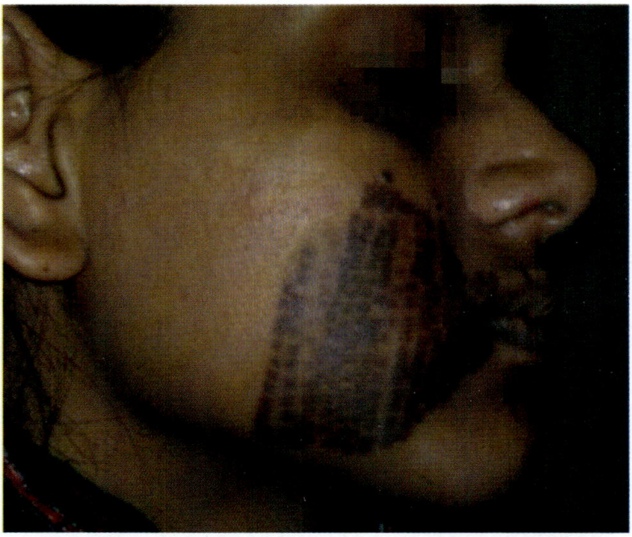

Fig. 4.17: Post-inflammatory hyperpigmentation in a female undergoing Q switched Nd YAG laser therapy

Cosmetic Camouflage

- Camouflage can be a useful alternative in patients with recalcitrant melasma and in situations requiring short term masking of lesions for social or professional reasons and can significantly improve the quality of life of the patients.
- Camouflage agents come in cream, compact, liquid or stick formulations.
- Ideal camouflage should be waterproof, non-translucent and long lasting agent with appropriate color blending and color corrections.

Suggested Readings

1. Chang MW; *Disorders of Hyperpigmentation,* In: Bolognia JL, Jorizzo JL, Schaffer JV, eds.; *Dermatology,* 3rd edn., Elsevier Saunders 2009, pp.1052-54.
2. Anstey AV; *Disorders of Skin Colour,* In: Burns T, Breathnach S, C Neil, Griffiths C, eds.; *Rook's Textbook of Dermatology,* 8th edn., Wiley-Blackwell 2010, pp. 58-34.
3. Lahiri K, Chatterjee M, Sarkar R, eds.; *Pigmentary Disorders, A Comprehensive Compendium,* New Delhi: Jaypee Brothers Medical Publishers (P) Ltd; 2014.
4. Sarkar R, Chugh S, Garg VK; *Newer and Upcoming Therapies for Melasma*; *Indian J Dermatol Venereol Leprol* 2012; 78: pp. 417-28.
5. Sheth VM, Pandya AG; *Melasma: A Comprehensive Update, Part I and II*; *J Am Acad Dermatol* 2011;65: pp. 689-714.
6. Sarkar R, Arora P, Garg VK, Sonthalia S, Gokhale N; *Melasma Update; Indian Dermatol Online* J 2014;5: pp. 426-35.
7. Sarkar R, Gupta AR, Sardana K; *Melasma,* In: *Diagnosis and Management of Skin Disorders; An Evidence-based Approach;* Sardana K, Garg VK, Mahajan S, eds., New Delhi, Wolters Kluwer Pvt Ltd 2012, pp. 543-50.

5 Hyperpigmentary Disorders Other Than Melasma

Lalit K Gupta, Nidheesh Agarwal, Manisha Balai, Urvashi Goyal

Chapter At A Glance

- **Hyperpigmentary disorders are common and often associated with significant psychosocial impact.**
- **Hyperpigmentation may result from either an increase in melanin production or from an increase in density of active melanocytes. It may also result from deposition of exogenous substances such as drugs or heavy metals within the dermis.**
- **Pigment excess in the epidermis imparts brownish hue while increased pigment in the dermis appears slate-gray to bluish-gray due to optical effect (Tyndall phenomenon). Recognition that pigment is epidermal or dermal helps to predict the treatment outcome.**
- **Several morphological patterns of pigmentation including linear, reticulate, flagellate, splashed, rippled, whorled, Blaschkoid and serpentine are recognized and provide vital clue to the diagnoses.**
- **Freckles, lentigines, post-inflammatory, macular amyloidosis, friction, nutritional deficiency, drugs and nevi are some of the common causes of hyperpigmentation.**
- **The management of hyperpigmentary disorders involves identification of etiological factors, photo protection and use of bleaching agents. Procedures like chemical peeling and lasers may be helpful in selected patients.**

INTRODUCTION

- Hyperpigmentary disorders may result from either hypermelanosis or deposition of exogenous substances such as drugs, drug complexes or heavy metals within the dermis.
- Hypermelanosis may be either epidermal, dermal or mixed, which may result from increase in number of melanocytes or their increased biological activity.
- The color of the lesions gives some clue to its location in the skin. Epidermal pigmentation is light brown to dark brown in color whereas dermal pigmentation is slate-gray to bluish-gray.
- Identification of this color difference is useful for treatment outcome as epidermal pigmentation is likely to respond better to treatment as compared to dermal pigmentation.
- **Dyschromatosis:** Characterized by the presence of both hypo- and hyperpigmentation (e.g. dyschromatosis symmetrica hereditaria).

CLASSIFICATION

- There is no uniform way to classify these disorders and the most practical approach for classification is shown in Box 5.1.

Box 5.1: Classification of hyperpigmentary disorders

Melanocytic (Increased number of melanocytes)
- **Epidermal**
  - Lentigines
- **Dermal**
  - Mongolian spot
  - Nevus of Ota/Ito
  - Nevus of Hori
  - Phakomatosis pigmentovascularis
  - Melanoma

Melanotic (Increased activity of melanocytes)
- **Epidermal**
  - Freckles
  - Café-au-lait macules

Contd.

Contd.

- Becker's nevus
- Nevus spilus
- Nutritional

- **Dermal**
  - Post-inflammatory hyperpigmentation
  - Drug induced and fixed drug eruption
  - Melasma
  - Macular amyloidosis
  - Pigmented contact dermatitis
  - Lichen planus pigmentosus
  - Ochronosis
  - Incontinentia pigmenti
  - Erythema dyschromicum perstans

Some of these conditions can be diagnosed due to their characteristic shapes and patterns as shown in Table 5.1.

Table 5.1: Characteristic patterns of some hyperpigmentary diseases

Pattern	Condition
Linear	Pigmentary demarcation lines
Reticulate	Reticulate acropigmentation of Kitamura, Dyskeratosis congenita
Flagellate	Bleomycin, Mushroom dermatitis
Splashed	Becker's nevus
Whorled	Linear and whorled nevoid hypermelanosis
Blaschkoid	Incontinentia pigmenti
Rippled	Macular amyloidosis
Serpentine	Dactinomycin, Vincristine

MELANOCYTIC HYPERPIGMENTATION

Lentiginosis

- Lentigo (plural: lentiginosis) is a Latin word that means a lentil-shaped pigmented macule.
- *Lentigo simplex* presents as well circumscribed, light-brown to dark-brown, homogenously pigmented macules measuring less than 5 mm in diameter occurring anywhere in the body, including mucosae without any predilection for sun exposed area (Fig. 5.1).

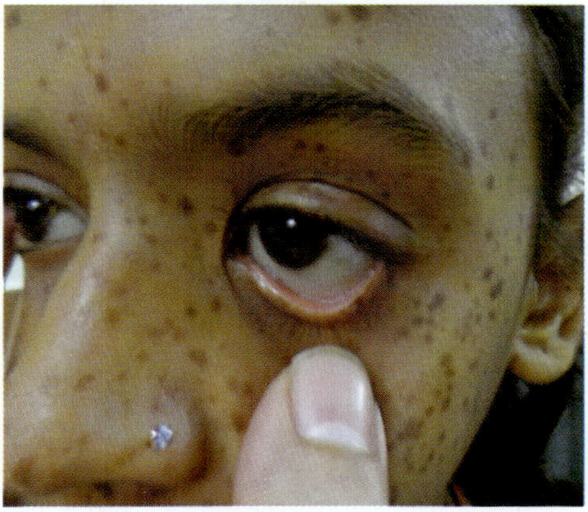

Fig. 5.1: Lentigines present over face and conjunctival mucosa

- *Solar lentigines* (Liver spots/Senile freckles) are characterized by well-circumscribed, dark brown or black, round, oval or irregularly shaped macules predominantly on sun-exposed areas and vary in size from about 3 mm to 2 cm (Fig. 5.2).They are more commonly seen in elderly and fair skinned individuals.

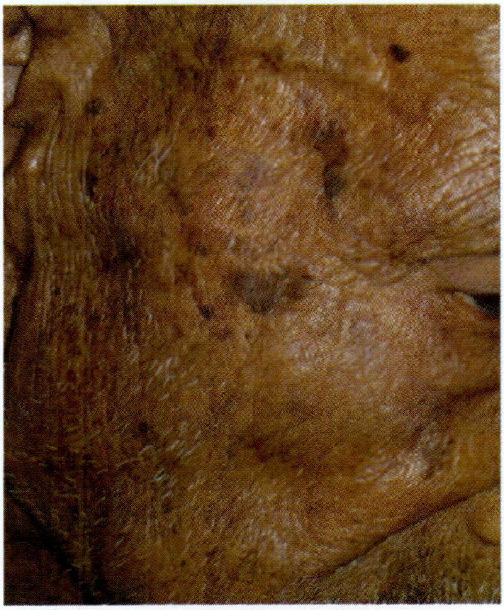

Fig. 5.2: Solar lentigines on the face of an elderly

- Lentigines may occur in isolation or can be associated with some syndromes (Table 5.2).

Table 5.2: Syndromes associated with lentiginosis

Disorders	Features
Centrofacial lentiginosis	• Lentigines in a butterfly distribution on the nose, cheeks>forehead, eyelids, upper lip • Neuropsychiatric features
LEOPARD (Moynahan) syndrome	• Generalized distribution of **L**entigines • **E**CG changes (conduction defects, hypertrophic cardiomyopathy), **O**cular hypertelorism, **P**ulmonary stenosis, **A**bnormal genitalia, growth **R**etardation and **D**eafness
Peutz-Jeghers syndrome	• Lentigines favor perioral region, oral mucosa and hands (Fig. 5.3) • Multiple hamartomatous gastrointestinal polyps with risk for malignancies
Cronkhite-Canada syndrome	• Lentigines of buccal mucosa, face, hands/feet • Alopecia (diffuse, non-scarring), nail dystrophy, intestinal polyposis
NAME syndrome	• **N**evi, **A**trial myxoma, **M**yxoid neurofibroma, **E**phelides
LAMB syndrome	• **L**entigines, **A**trial myxoma, **M**ucocutaneous myxoma, **B**lue nevi
Partial unilateral lentiginosis	• Multiple lentigines in a segmental distribution • Café-au-lait macules in same distribution

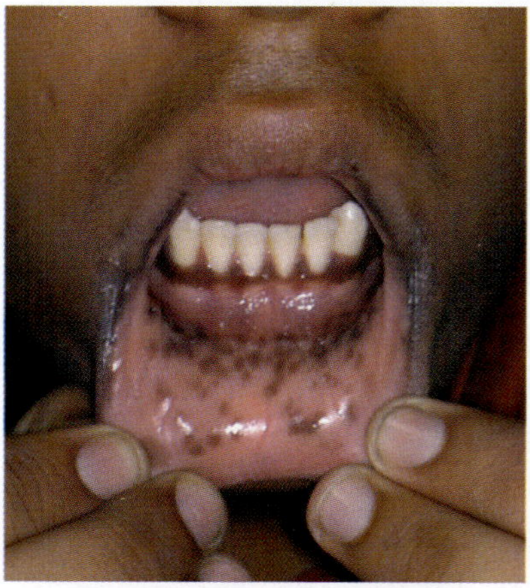

Fig. 5.3: Mucosal lentigines in Peutz-Jeghers syndrome

Mongolian Spots (Congenital Dermal Melanocytosis)

- A common condition characterized by blue to bluish-grey patches over sacrococcygeal/lumbar region and buttocks, usually present since birth and regress during early childhood (Fig. 5.4).
- Size varies from few cms to more than 10 cms.

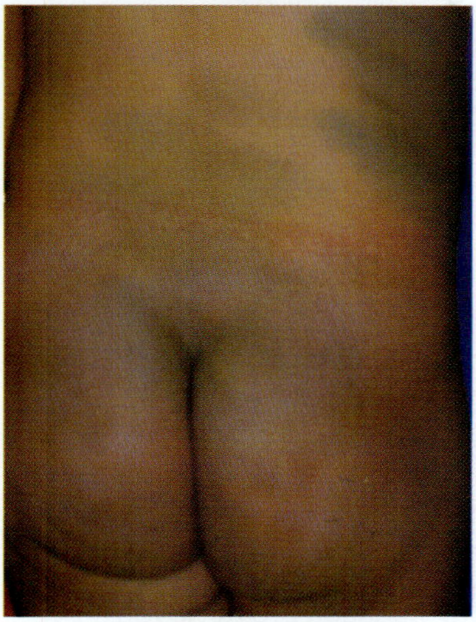

Fig. 5.4: Mongolian spots

Nevus of Ota (Nevus Fuscoceruleus Ophthalmomaxillaris)

- Onset is bimodal, with half of the cases having onset before the age of 1 year and in another half around puberty; more common in females.
- Characterized by ill-defined, blue-grey pigmented macules on the face along the ophthalmic and maxillary branches of trigeminal nerve. Associated scleral pigmentation may aid in the diagnosis (Fig. 5.5a,b).
- Lesions are usually unilateral (Fig. 5.5a) but bilateral involvement (Fig. 5.5b) may be seen in 5% cases.

Nevus of Ito

- Clinically similar to nevus of Ota but present over supraclavicular,

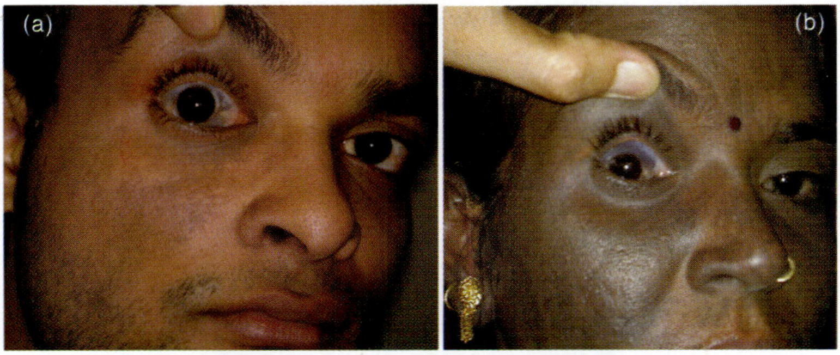

Fig. 5.5: Nevus of Ota. Typical slate gray pigmentation on face unilaterally (Fig. 5.5a). Bilateral nevus of Ota (Fig. 5.5b) is relatively uncommon. Note the typical scleral pigmentation in both the pictures

scapular and deltoid regions which are innervated by posterior supraclavicular and lateral brachiocutaneous nerves.

Nevus of Hori (Acquired Bilateral Nevus of Ota like Macules)

- Characterized by bilateral blue-brown or slate gray macules over zygomatic area.
- Ocular and oral mucosae are not involved.
- May be confused with melasma due to its bilateral distribution.

Phakomatosis Pigmentovascularis

- Phakomatosis refers to a developmental malformation simultaneously affecting the eye, skin and central nervous system.
- Characterized by presence of nevus flammeus with pigmentary nevi of various types like nevus of Ota, nevus spilus, Mongolian spots, nevus depigmentosus and nevus anemicus.
- Five types have been described, of which type II (nevus flammeus + dermal melanocytosis +/-nevus anemicus) is the most common form (Fig. 5.6).
- In the lesions on face, ruling out of Sturge-Weber syndrome is important.

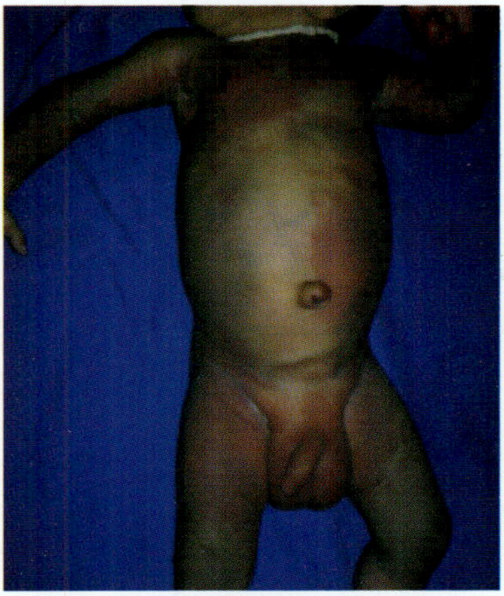

Fig. 5.6: Phakomatosis pigmentovascularis

MELANOTIC HYPERPIGMENTATION

Freckles (Ephelides)

- Characterized by small, 2-4 mm sized well-circumscribed, light brown macules over sun-exposed areas commonly in individuals with fair skin (Fig. 5.7).

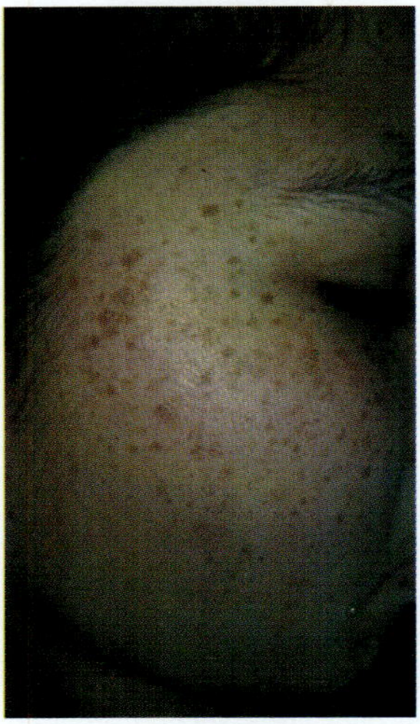

Fig. 5.7: Freckles in a fair skinned female

- Not present at birth, but usually appear during the first 3 years of life.
- They may be cosmetically disfiguring.
- May be confused with lentigines, but can be clinically distinguished by features described in Table 5.3.

Table 5.3: Distinguishing features between freckles and lentigines

	Freckles	Lentigines
Color	Light brown	Light to dark brown
Distribution	Sun exposed	No such predilection
Duration of lesions	Fade with photoprotection	Persist for life
Seasonal variation	Darken in summers, fade in winters and with ageing	May darken in summers but do not fade in winters
Histopathology	Increased melanocyte activity	Increased melanocyte number

- Widespread freckling, starting at an early age, predominantly over sun exposed sites and with a tendency to develop malignancy is a feature of xeroderma pigmentosum due to DNA instability and excision repair defect (Fig. 5.8).

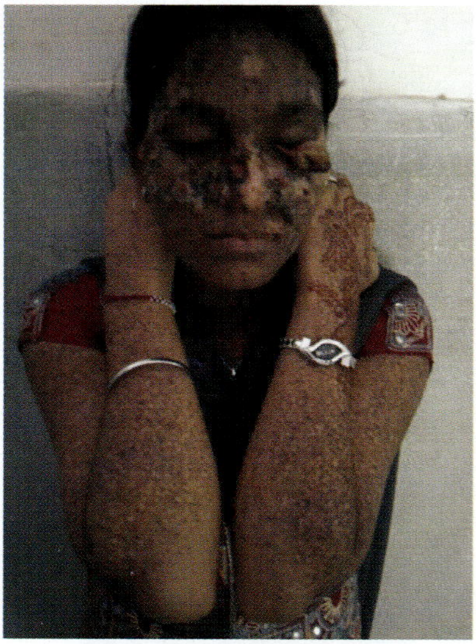

Fig. 5.8: Extensive freckling over sun exposed areas in a patient of xeroderma pigmentosum. Also notice the cutaneous malignancies over face

Café-au-lait Macules (CALMs)

- Homogenously brown colored well defined macules, varying in size from 0.5 cm to more than 20 cms (Fig. 5.9).

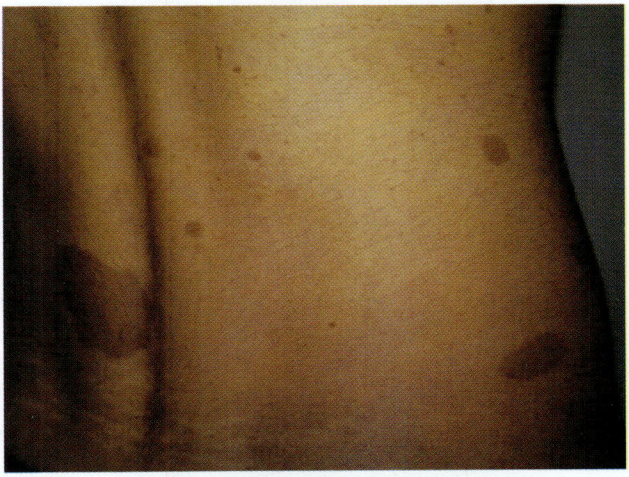

Fig. 5.9: Café-au-lait macules

- May be present at birth or appear in the early months of life.
- Isolated CALMs can be a physiological finding in about 10-20% of the normal population.
- Commonly distributed over trunk and buttocks; head and neck are usually spared.
- Numerous and large CALMs indicate multisystem involvement and association with some syndromes (Table 5.4).

Becker's Nevus (Pigmented Hairy Epidermal Nevus)

- Onset is usually during the second or third decade of life and is more common in males than in females.
- It is characterized by irregular macular hyperpigmentation on shoulder, anterior chest or scapular region (Fig. 5.10). The lesions have a typical splashed appearance and may develop hypertrichosis and acneiform lesions with time.

Table 5.4: Disorders associated with multiple CALMs

Disorders	Features
Neurofibromatosis 1	6 or more CALMs, Crowe's sign (skin fold freckling), neurofibromas, optic glioma, skeletal dysplasia
Neurofibromatosis 2	Acoustic neuromas, schwannomas, meningiomas
Legius (NF1-like) syndrome	6 or more CALMs, intertriginous freckling
McCune-Albright syndrome	Segmental CALMs, polyostotic fibrous dysplasia, precocious puberty
LEOPARD syndrome	Café noir, lentigines, cardiac conduction defects, ocular hypertelorism, pulmonary stenosis, growth retardation, hearing loss
Cowden syndrome	Multiple trichilemmomas, cobblestoning of oral mucosa, palmoplantar keratosis, hamartomas and carcinoma of breast, thyroid, colon
Tuberous sclerosis	Mental retardation, seizures, hypopigmented macules, CALMs, angiofibromas
Fanconi anemia	Hyperpigmented macules, pancytopenia, multiple congenital anomalies, chromosomal fragility and malignancies

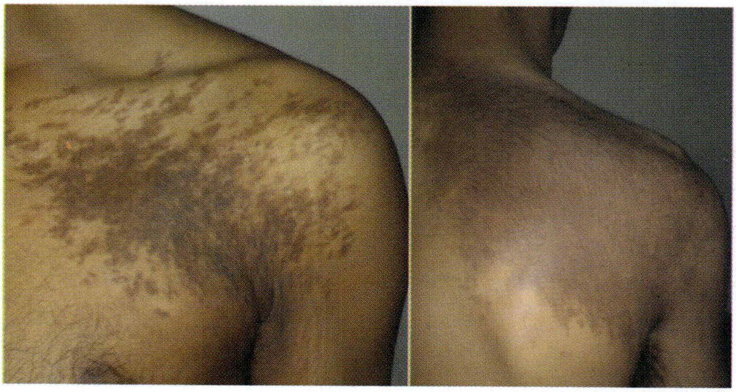

Fig. 5.10: Becker's nevus. Notice the typical splashed appearance and hypertrichosis

- Ipsilateral developmental abnormalities such as breast hypoplasia and supernumery nipples, aplasia of pectoralis major muscle, limb reduction may be associated.

Nevus Spilus (Speckled Lentiginous Nevus)

- Presents as circumscribed, pigmented macule or patch with superimposed "speckles" which consist of scattered more darkly pigmented lentigo-like lesions that may increase with time (Fig. 5.11).

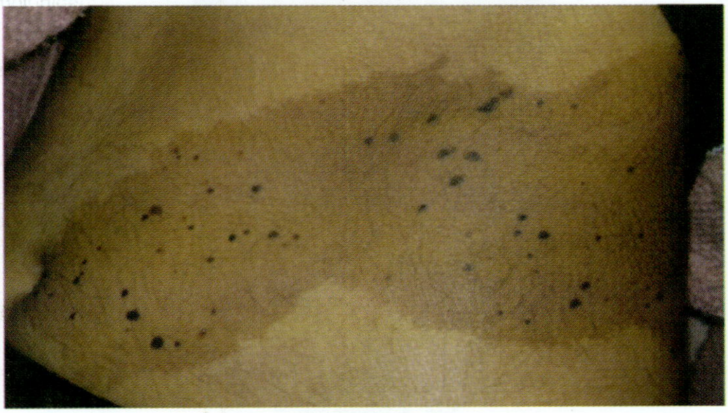

Fig. 5.11: Nevus spilus

Nutritional Disorders

Nutritional deficiency is an important but under reported cause of hyperpigmentation, especially in the Indian scenario. Coexistent deficiencies of multiple nutrients usually occur, and it may not be possible to attribute the hyperpigmentation to a specific deficiency; however, a few patterns have been recognized:

- **Vitamin B_{12} deficiency:** Generalized deep brown to brownish-black pigmentation, more prominent in the creases of palms and fingers and on knuckles. Pigmentation of nail bed and finger tips may be seen.
- **Folic acid deficiency:** Diffuse or localized greyish-brown pigmentation on sun-exposed areas.
- **Vitamin B_3 deficiency (Pellagra):** Addisonian type hyperpigmentation with involvement of face, hands and areas of friction and pressure is seen during active disease. Also, skin lesions of pellagroid dermatitis may leave behind PIH (Fig. 5.12).
- **Vitamin A deficiency:** Generalized pigmentation with hyperpigmentation of horny follicular papules.

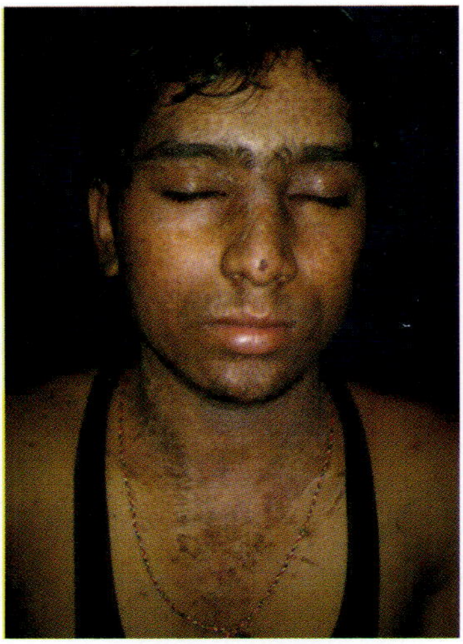

Fig. 5.12: Pellagra

- **Vitamin C deficiency:** Perifollicular discoloration on legs and sometimes Addisonian type pigmentation may present.
- **Malabsorption syndromes:** Addisonian type hyperpigmentation, with (Fig. 5.13) or without mucosal involvement, may be seen in sprue and other malabsorption syndromes.

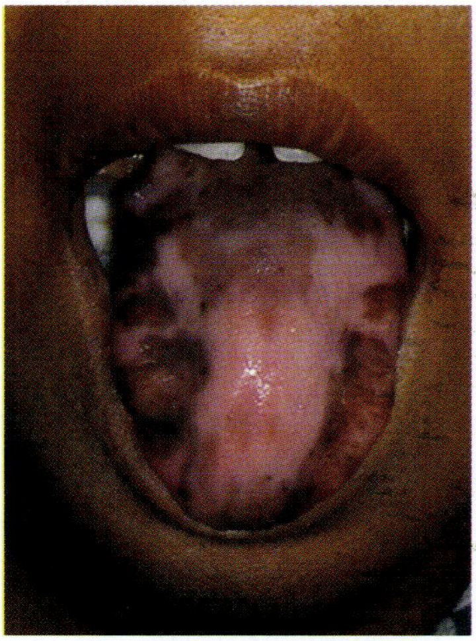

Fig. 5.13: Mucosal pigmentation due to nutritional deficiency

Post-Inflammatory Hyperpigmentation (PIH)

- Perhaps the most common cause of hyperpigmentation and represents an excess of pigment following cutaneous inflammation or injury, anywhere on the skin surface, including the mucous membranes and the nail unit.
- Dark-skinned persons (Fitzpatrick skin types III to VI) tend to have a greater frequency, severity and duration of PIH than those with lighter complexions.
- Various factors determining the character of pigmentation are:
  - Depth of pigment (brown-epidermal location; bluish gray-dermal location).
  - Degree of inflammation.
  - Causative inflammatory disease.
- PIH can be exacerbated by continued inflammation, trauma or exposure to ultraviolet irradiation.
- Epidermal PIH generally resolves over time, although fading may require months or years in darkly pigmented individuals. Dermal PIH tends to persist longer and is sometimes permanent.
- Common dermatoses which heal with PIH are shown in Box 5.2.

Box 5.2: Dermatoses with post-inflammatory hyperpigmentation (Figs. 5.14 to 5.23)

- Dermatitis (irritant/allergic contact, photocontact, atopic dermatitis)
- Inflammatory dermatoses (acne vulgaris, fixed drug eruption, lichen planus, psoriasis, lupus erythematosus, insect bites)
- Immunobullous diseases (pemphigus, bullous pemphigoid)
- Infectious diseases (pyoderma, dermatophytoses, herpes zoster)
- Iatrogenic (retinoids, chemical peels, lasers, microdermabrasion)

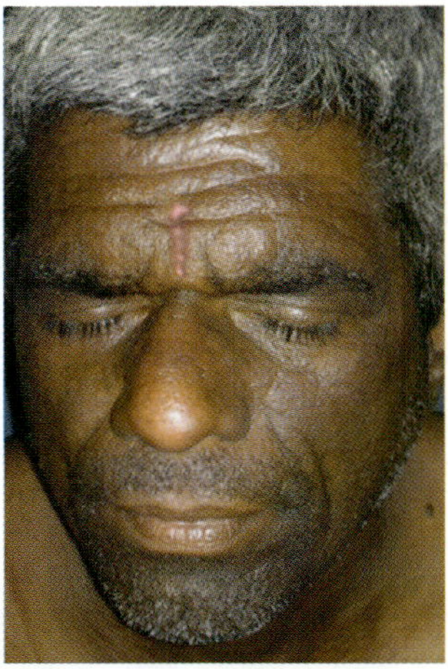

Fig. 5.14: PIH secondary to air borne contact dermatitis

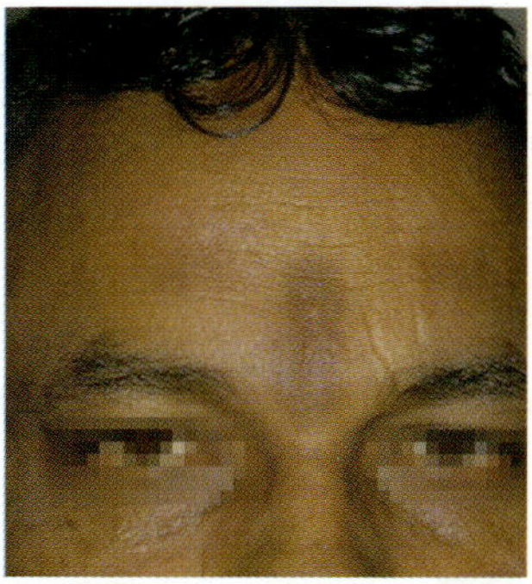

Fig. 5.15: PIH secondary to allergic contact dermatitis due to application of "tika"

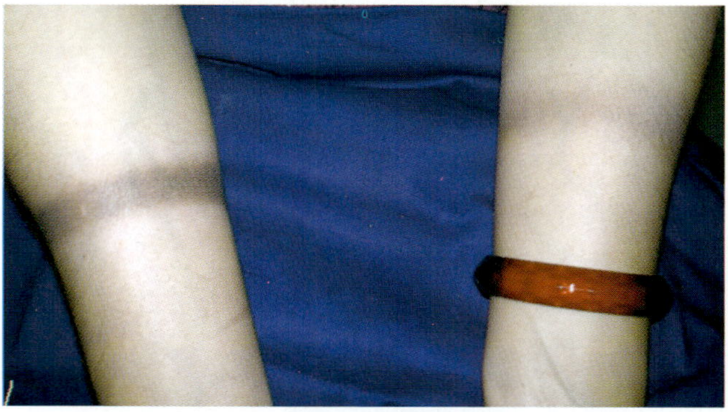

Fig. 5.16: PIH secondary to allergic contact dermatitis due to bangles

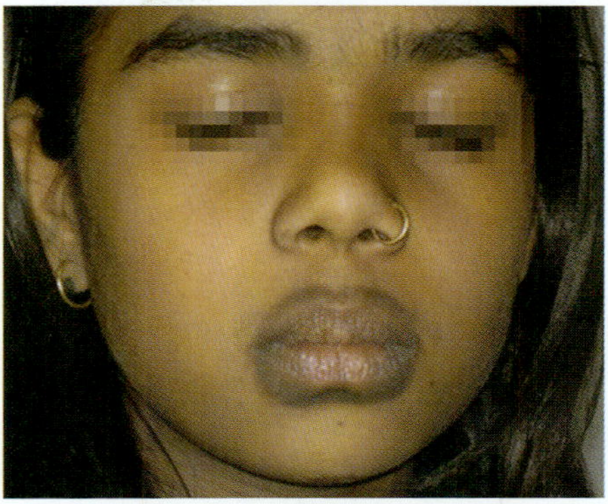

Fig. 5.17: PIH secondary to lip licking dermatitis. The patient had an atopic diathesis

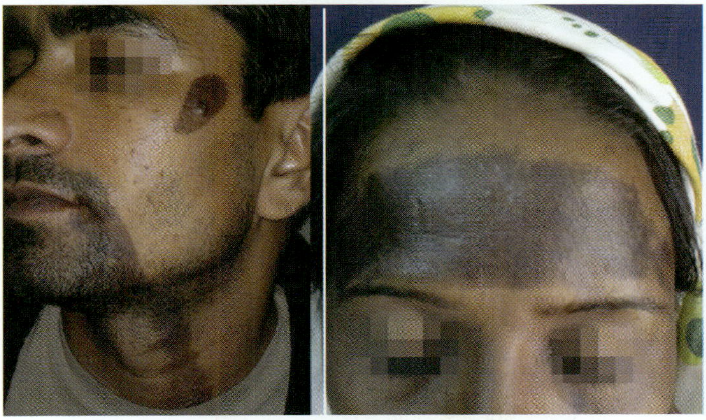

Fig. 5.18: PIH secondary to irritant contact dermatitis

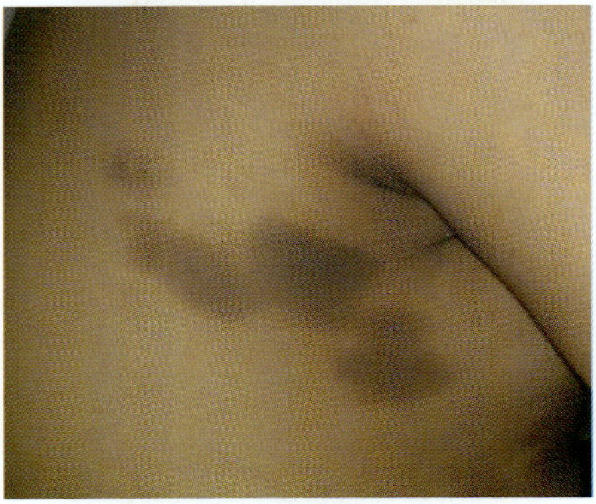

Fig. 5.19: PIH due to fixed drug eruption

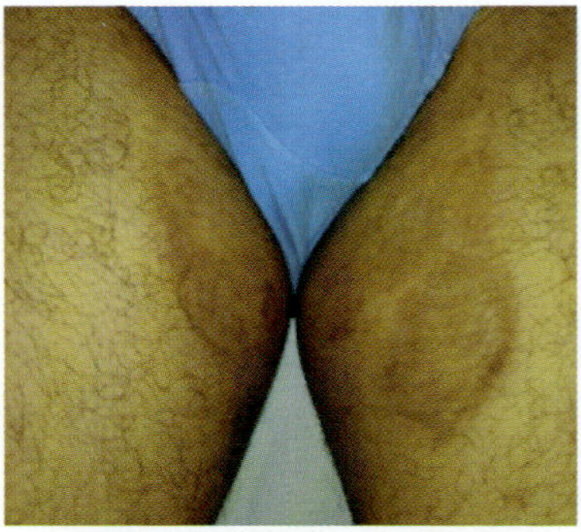

Fig. 5.20: PIH secondary to tinea cruris

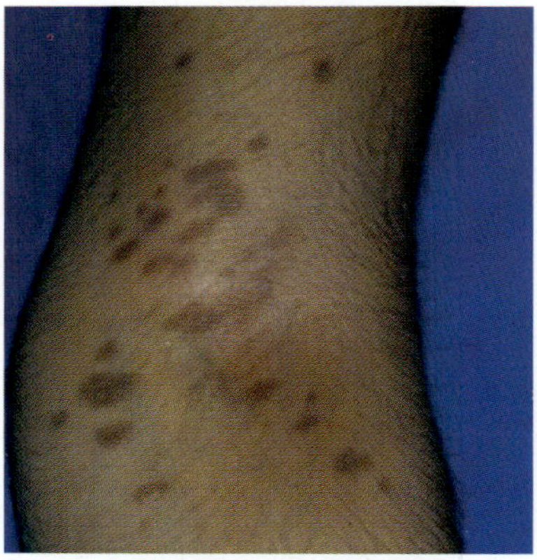

Fig. 5.21: PIH due to lichen planus

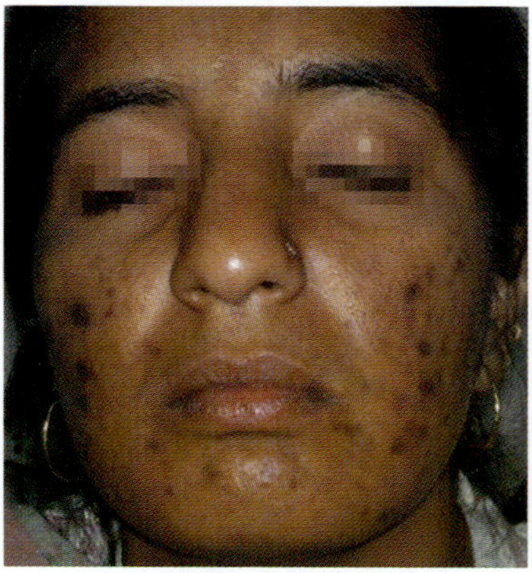

Fig. 5.22: PIH secondary to acne vulgaris

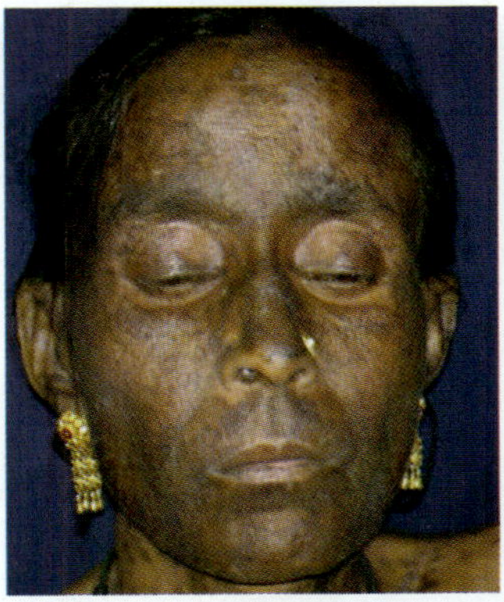

Fig. 5.23: PIH in a patient of systemic lupus erythematosus

Drug Induced Hypermelanosis

- Hyperpigmentation of the skin (localized or generalized) may be caused by several drugs through various mechanisms. Commonly used drugs which cause hyperpigmentation are shown in Table 5.5.

Table 5.5: Clinical features of drugs causing hypermelanosis	
Drug	**Clinical features**
Clofazimine	• Diffuse reddish-brown discoloration of skin (Fig. 5.24). • Pigmentation is due to high lipophilicity of drug.
Zidovudine	• Longitudinal/transverse and diffuse melanonychia along with mucocutaneous hyperpigmentation (Fig. 5.25).
Anti-malarials (Chloroquine, Hydroxychloroquine)	• Gray to blue-black pigmentation over face and pretibial areas, hard palate, sclera and subungual areas. • Pigmentation may be due to drug-melanin complex.
Minocycline	• Those with higher cumulative dose (> 100 g) may develop hyperpigmentation over sun-exposed areas, sites of prior inflammation and scars, anterior shins and arms. • May also involve nails, sclera, oral mucosa, bones, thyroid, breast and teeth.
Bleomycin	• Linear, flagellate bands that favor the trunk. • Transverse melanonychia.
Amiodarone	• Blue-grey to violaceous discoloration of sun-exposed skin, especially face.
Psychotropic drugs	• Blue or slate-grey discoloration in sun-exposed areas.
Psoralens	• Diffuse or circumscribed hyperpigmentation seen with oral and topical psoralens respectively.

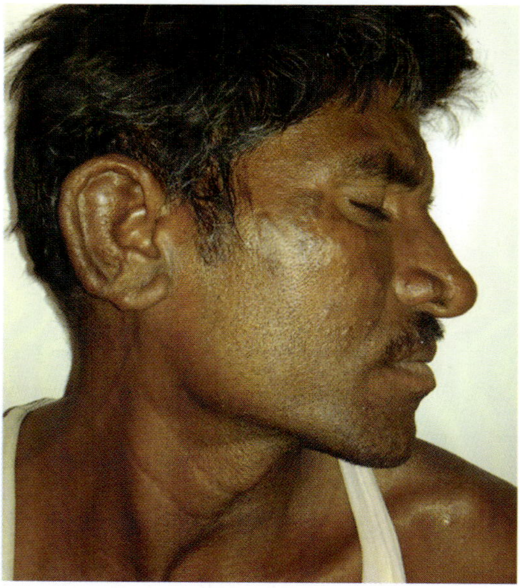

Fig. 5.24: Clofazimine induced pigmentation in a patient of lepromatous leprosy

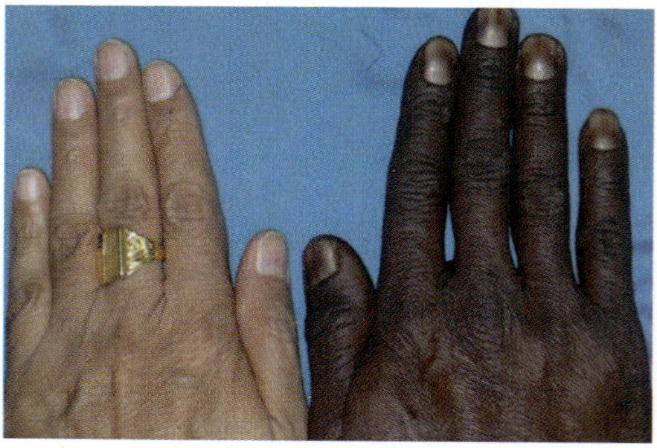

Fig. 5.25: Zidovudine induced pigmentation of skin and nails and its comparison with normal skin color

- Heavy metals (arsenic, bismuth, gold, mercury, silver), chemotherapeutic agents (cyclophoshamide, 5-Fluorouracil, busulphan, doxorubicin, hydroxyurea), oral contraceptives, epidermal growth factor receptor inhibitor may also cause hyperpigmentation.

Fixed Drug Eruption

- A common pattern of drug reaction, characterized by development of one or more annular or oval erythematous patches/plaques (Fig. 5.26), which develop 30 min to 8 hours following drug administration and heal with intense hyperpigmentation (Fig. 5.19).

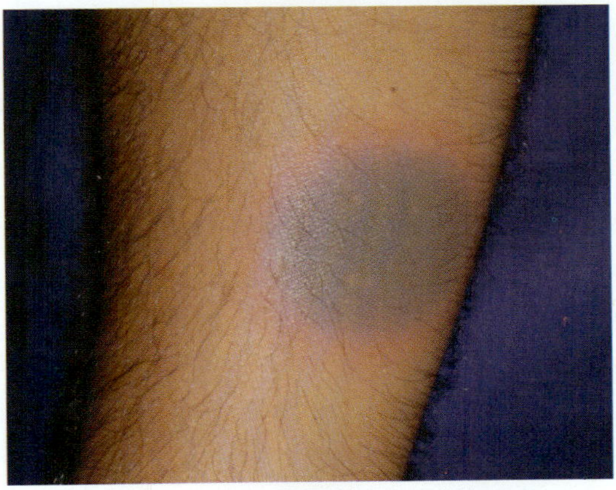

Fig. 5.26: Classical lesion of fixed drug eruption

- The lesions recur at exactly the same site(s) with each subsequent exposure to the drug.
- Hands, feet, face and mucosae are favored sites.
- Most commonly implicated drugs are trimethoprim-sulfamethoxazole, imidazoles (metronidazole, tinidazole, ornidazole), tetracyclines, and nonsteroidal anti-inflammatory drugs.

Macular Amyloidosis

- Presents as brown to gray-brown hyperpigmentation in a characteristic reticulate or "rippled" pattern, predominantly over interscapular area (Fig. 5.27).
- Often pruritic and rubbing plays a key role in the development of lesions.
- Histopathology is characteristic and shows amyloid deposition confined to papillary dermis that exhibits green birefringence with Congo red when viewed under polarizing microscope.

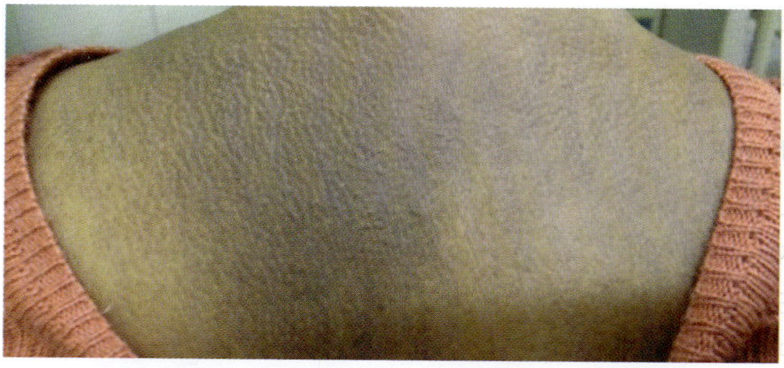

Fig. 5.27: Macular amyloidosis. Notice the rippled pigmentation in interscapular area

Riehl's Melanosis (Pigmented Cosmetic/Contact Dermatitis)

- Presumed to be caused by repeated exposure of allergens present in cosmetics (aniline and azo dyes, hair dyes, red kumkum, fragrances etc.) and textiles (optical whiteners, dyes, formaldehyde etc.).
- In India, kumkum and hair dyes are most common allergens.
- Clinically characterized by diffuse, patchy or reticular pigmentation on face (cosmetics) as seen in Fig. 5.28 and anterior aspect of thighs and axillae (textiles).

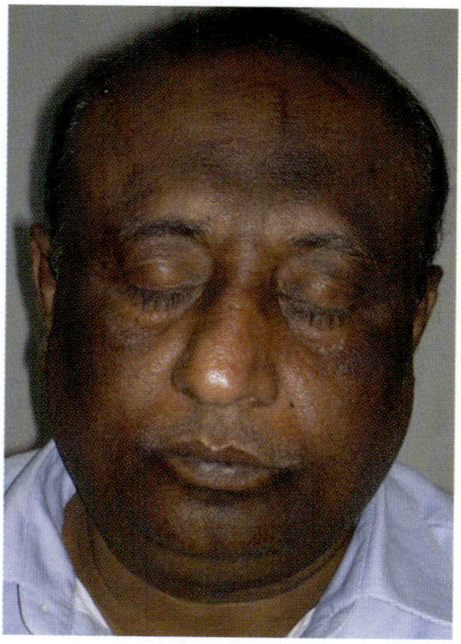

Fig. 5.28: Riehl's melanosis

- Patch test and photopatch test can be helpful in finding the allergens.

Lichen Planus Pigmentosus (LPP)

- LPP is a chronic macular variant of lichen planus that favors young to middle-aged adults with skin phototypes III-V.
- Etiology is unknown. Possible risk factors are sun exposure, use of mustard oil and amla oil for body massage/hair dressing and chronic use of henna or hair dyes.
- Presents as asymptomatic gray-brown to dark brown pigmented macules and patches initially over sun exposed areas especially the forehead, temples and neck and later involving the covered parts (Fig. 5.29).

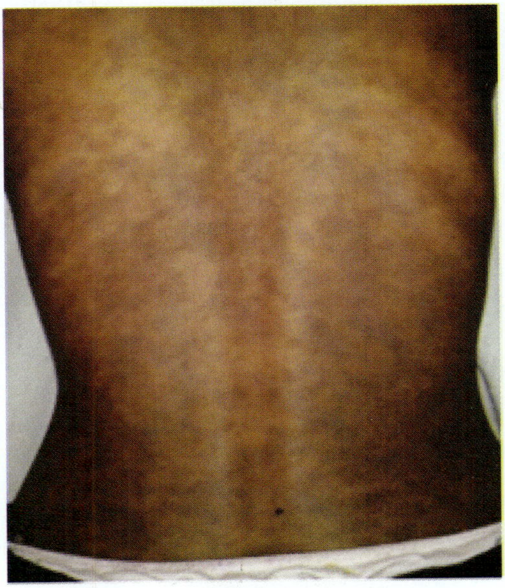

Fig. 5.29: Grayish brown lesions of LPP on trunk

- A close differential diagnosis is erythema dyschromicum perstans (EDP) or ashy dermatoses which can be differentiated based on the features shown in Table 5.6.

Table 5.6: Differences between LPP and EDP

	LPP	EDP
Sex	M=F	F>M
Age	Childhood to old age	3rd - 4th decade
Border	Not raised	Characteristic raised thready border
Reticulate pattern	+/-	-
Distribution	Non-characteristic	Symmetrical
Areas	Sun-exposed and flexural areas	Trunk, neck, face, upper limbs
Pruritus	+/-	-

Ochronosis

- Two forms seen: Exogenous and endogenous.
- Exogenous is more common, localized over face and results from paradoxical hyperpigmentation following chronic use of hydroquinone (Figs. 4.15 and 4.16).
- Endogenous is due to accumulation of homogentisic acid (alkaptonuria).
- Pigment is deposited throughout the skin but is more apparent over joints, tympanic membrane, thenar and hypothenar eminences, sides of fingers and ear cartilage.
- Histologically characteristic yellow-brown banana-shaped bodies are seen in papillary dermis.

PATTERNED HYPERPIGMENTATION

Linear Hyperpigmentation

- Can have a variety of causes like post-inflammatory, drug reactions and mosaic genetic alterations that result in hypermelanosis along the lines of Blaschko.

Pigmentary Demarcation Lines (Futcher's Lines, Voigt's Lines, Ito's Lines)

- Physiological, more prominent in darker skin types, bilaterally symmetrical lines that probably mark the abrupt transition between deeper and lighter pigmented skin.

- Most common on the anterolateral upper arm and posteromedial thigh.
- Different patterns and clinical features of pigmentary demarcation lines have been described in Table 5.7.

Table 5.7: Patterns of pigmentary demarcation lines

Types	Description
A	Vertical line along the lateral aspect of upper arm extending over the pectoral area
B	Curved line on the posteromedial thigh that extends from the perineum to the popliteal fossa (Fig. 5.30)
C	Mediosternal line, a vertical hypopigmented line in the pre and parasternal area
D	A vertical line in a pre- or paraspinal location
E	Bilateral hypopigmented streaks, bands or lanceolate areas over the chest in a zone that runs from the mid third of the clavicle to the periareolar skin
F	"V" shaped hyperpigmented lines between the malar prominence and the temple
G	"W" shaped hyperpigmented lines between the malar prominence and the temple
H	Linear bands of hyperpigmentation from the angle of mouth to lateral aspect of chin

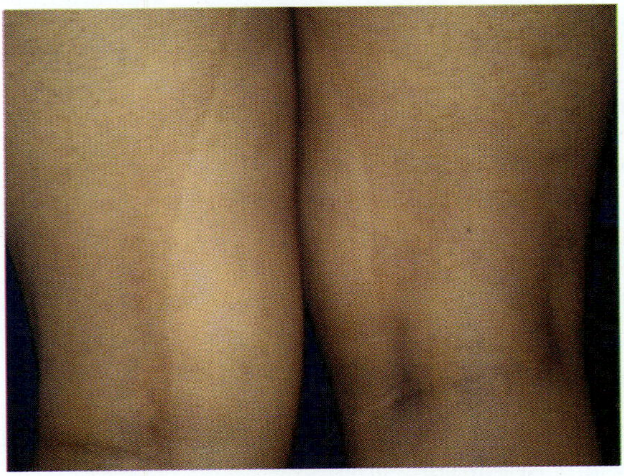

Fig. 5.30: Type B pigmentary demarcation lines seen on thighs during pregnancy

Linear Post-Inflammatory Hyperpigmentation

- As a result of healed linear dermatoses like blister beetle dermatitis, poison ivy dermatitis, linear lichen planus, linear psoriasis, chemical phlebitis etc.

Flagellate Pigmentation (Scratch Dermatitis)

- Most commonly due to bleomycin, seen in 10-20% of patients, 1-9 weeks after administration of the drug, usually after a cumulative dose of 100-300 mg.
- As a result of microtrauma from scratching and drug-induced local increase in melanogenesis or alteration of pigment maturation.
- Characterized by asymptomatic or mildly itchy linear erythemato-violaceous streaks on the trunk and shoulder, followed by hyper-pigmentation.
- Flagellate mushroom dermatitis seen in individuals who have ingested large amounts of raw shiitake mushrooms or in those who cultivate these mushrooms can closely mimic the condition.

Hyperpigmentation Along Lines of Blaschko

- Dermatoses that follow the lines of Blaschko resulting from mosaicism include 2 main entities namely *linear and whorled nevoid hypermelanosis* and *incontinentia pigmenti*.

Linear and Whorled Nevoid Hypermelanosis

- Characterized by swirls and streaks of macular hyperpigmentation along the lines of Blaschko that usually appear early during the first year of life and tend to persist indefinitely (Fig. 5.31).
- In some cases both hypo- and hyperpigmented streaks are simultaneously present, which may be referred to as "linear nevoid pigmentation".
- Up to a quarter of patients have associated neurologic, mus-culoskeletal or cardiac symptoms.

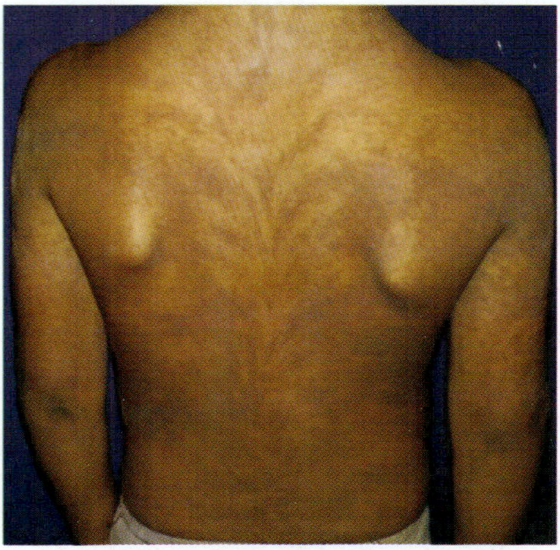

Fig. 5.31: Linear and whorled hypermelanosis

Incontinentia Pigmenti (Bloch-Sulzberger Syndrome)

- X-linked dominant multisystem disorder characterized by abnormalities of skin, teeth, hair and eyes.
- Most cases are female as the disease is lethal in males.
- The first stage is vesicobullous, or inflammatory stage with eosinophilia. In second stage pustular, verrucous and lichenoid lesions develop over limbs. The most characteristic is the third stage that shows gray to gray-brown streaks and whorls along the lines of Blaschko.
- The pigmentation fades gradually during late childhood to adolescence.

Reticulate Hyperpigmentation

- A clinical and genetically heterogenous group of disorders characterized by discrete or confluent freckle like hyperpigmented macules, arranged in a net like fashion. May be inherited or acquired.
- A condition with confusing nosology and often includes several interchangeable and overlapping terms like:
  - **Mottled:** Umbrella term for all disorders with variable hue, size and shape of pigmentation.

- **Dyschromatosis:** Both hypo and hyperpigmented macules of small size and irregular shapes.
- **Reticular:** Net like or lacy, regularly spaced lesions with areas of intervening normal skin.
- **Poikilodermatous:** Triad of atrophy, reticulate pigmentation and telangiectasias.

- Some of these disorders may have involvement of other ectodermal structures and may be associated with malignancies and life threatening systemic involvement.
- Clinical features of disorder with reticular pigmentation are shown in Table 5.8.

Table 5.8: Disorders characterized by reticular pigmentation

Disease	Features
Confluent and reticulated papillomatosis	• Characterized by asymptomatic, brown, hyperkeratotic, verrucous papules (Fig. 5.32) in inframammary, interscapular and epigastric regions • Responds well to minocycline
Prurigo pigmentosa	• Typically seen in young Japanese women • Characterized by recurrent crops of pruritic papulovesicles that resolve with a reticulated pattern of hyperpigmentation • Favored sites are back, neck and chest
Erythema ab igne	• Widely spaced net that corresponds to vascular pattern (Fig. 5.33) • Due to heat injury
Reticulate acropigmentation of Kitamura	• Reticulate, lentigo-like pigmentation on dorsal aspects of hands and feet (Fig. 5.34) • Small pits on palms and dorsum of fingers
Dyskeratosis congenita	• Fine, reticulate, grey-brown pigmentation on the neck and thighs • Atrophy of the skin, nail dystrophy and mucosal leucokeratosis of tongue
Dowling-Degos Disease (DDD)	• Reticulated hyperpigmentation of major flexures • Comedones on the back and neck • Pitted facial scars

Contd.

Contd.

Dermatopathia pigmentosa reticularis	• Persistent reticulated hyperpigmentation, alopecia, nail dystrophy • Palmoplantar keratoderma and hypoplastic dermatoglyphics in some patients
Naegeli-Franceschetti-Jadassohn syndrome	• Fading reticulated hyperpigmentation • Dental anomalies, hypohidrosis • Palmoplantar keratoderma, hypoplastic dermatoglyphics, nail dystrophy

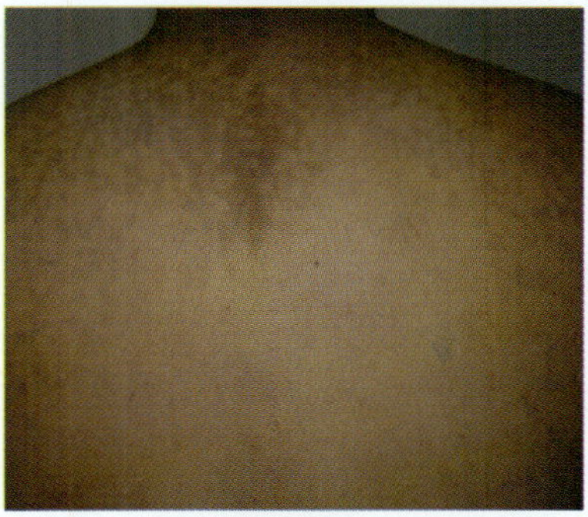

Fig. 5.32: Confluent and reticulated papillomatosis

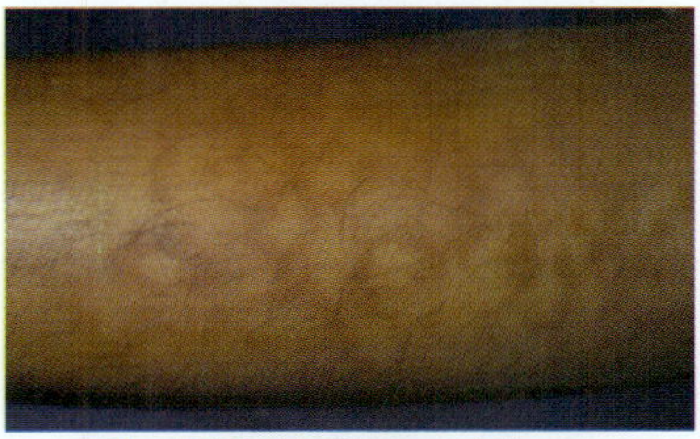

Fig. 5.33: Erythema ab igne

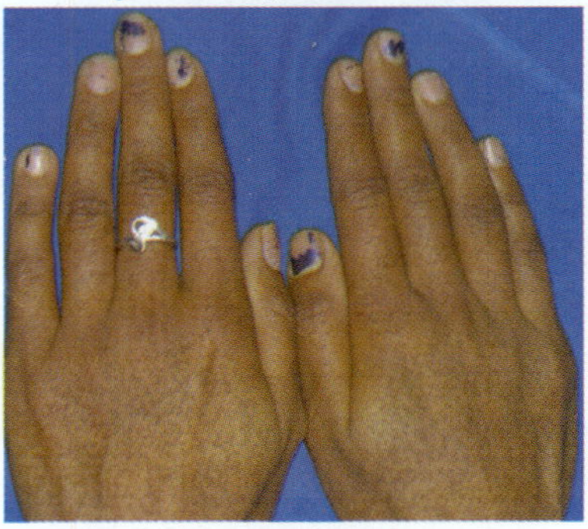

Fig. 5.34: Reticulate acropigmentation of Kitamura

FACIAL MELANOSES

- Facial melanoses other than melasma present with overlapping features and cause diagnostic and therapeutic difficulties. Some of these melanoses are shown in Box 5.3.

Box 5.3: Non-melasma facial melanoses
Acanthosis nigricans
Periorbital and perioral melanosis
Exogenous ochronosis
Pigmented contact dermatitis
Frictional melanosis
Lichen planus pigmentosus
Erythema dyschromicum perstans
Erythromelanosis follicularis faciei et colli

Acanthosis Nigricans

Characterized by hyperpigmented, verrucous or velvety plaques, on neck (Fig. 5.35), axillae, groin, other flexures and temples of face. Usually seen in obese, diabetics, and sometimes as a paraneoplastic condition.

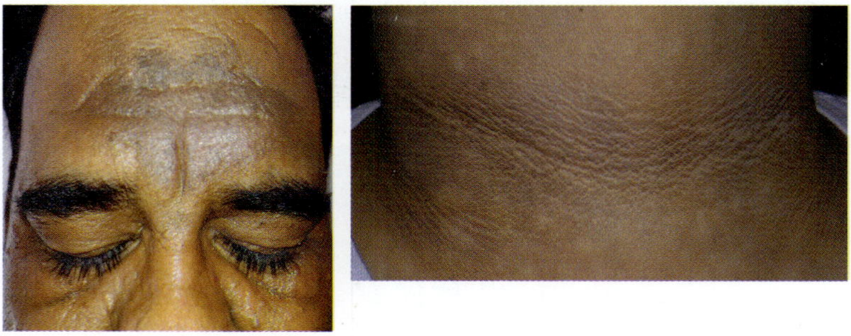

Fig. 5.35: Acanthosis nigricans

Periorbital Melanosis (Periocular Melanosis, Infraorbital Melanosis or Under Eye Dark Circles)

- A common condition causing great cosmetic concern.

- Characterized by brown to black pigmentation around the eyes bilaterally in middle aged individuals (Fig. 5.36) and believed to be an extension of pigmentary demarcation line type F of the face.

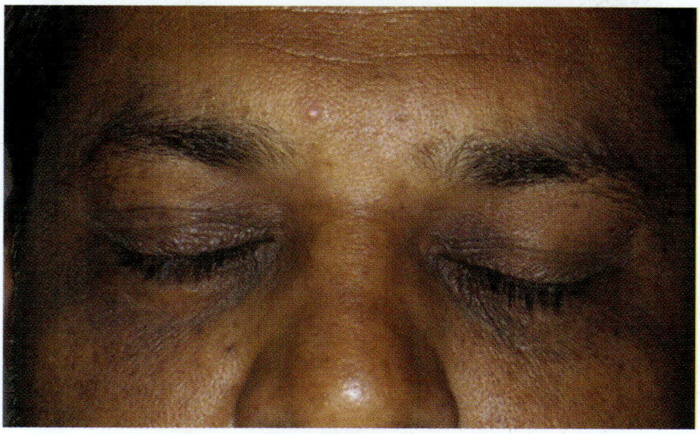

Fig. 5.36: Periorbital melanosis

- Exact etiology is not known but role of various endogenous and exogenous factors have been incriminated (Table 5.9).

Table 5.9: Factors incriminated in periorbital melanosis

Endogenous factors	Exogenous factors
• Genetics • Stress • Lack of sleep • Shadowing from lax skin • Superficial location of vasculature • Dermal melanin deposition • Infra orbital swelling	• PIH from atopic or allergic contact dermatitis • Use of lead of kohl pencils, cosmetics and ophthalmic solutions • Lifestyle factors such as excessive intake of caffeinated beverages

Erythromelanosis Follicularis Faciei et Colli

- The disorder is thought to be a variant of keratosis pilaris in pigmented skin, and is probably underreported in literature.
- Characterized by well-demarcated erythema, reddish-brown pigmentation, telangiectasia and tiny follicular papules on cheeks (Fig. 5.37), extending to side of neck, and/or extensor aspect of arms.

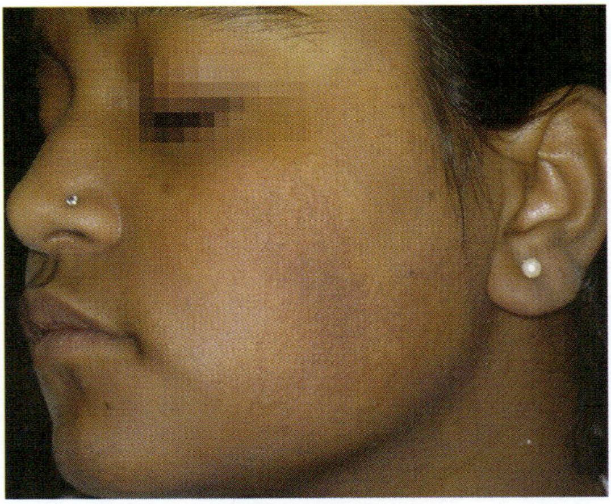

Fig. 5.37: Erythromelanosis follicularis faciei et colli

- Pigmentation spreads gradually and then become persistent and is refractory to treatment.

MISCELLANEOUS CAUSES OF HYPERPIGMENTATION

Addison's Disease

- Hyperpigmentation is almost universal in Addisonian patients.
- It is usually diffuse, and is most intense on light exposed areas, flexures, creases of palms and soles (Fig. 5.38), normally pigmented areas (nipples and genital skin) and sites of pressure.

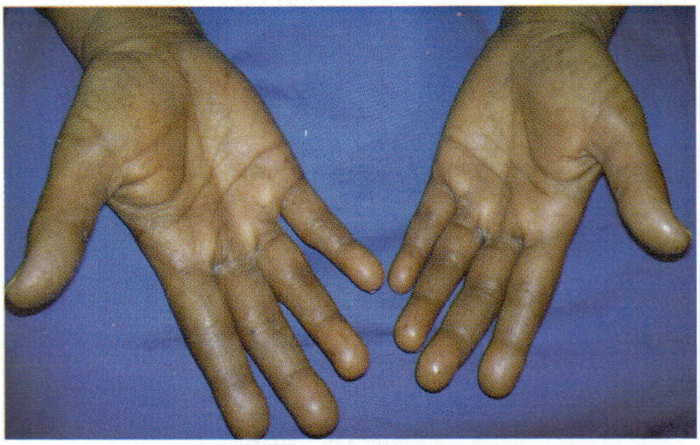

Fig. 5.38: Hyperpigmentation of palms and palmar creases in Addison's disease

- Pigmentation of the buccal and other mucosae may be present.
- Addisonian type of pigmentation may also be a feature of acromegaly, Cushing's syndrome, thyrotoxicosis and nutritional deficiencies.
- Pregnancy associated endocrinal changes may also lead to Addisonian type of hyperpigmentation.

Scleroderma and Morphea

- Diffuse or Addisonian type of pigmentation is seen in diffuse and localized scleroderma (morphea) as seen in (Figs. 5.39 and 5.40).

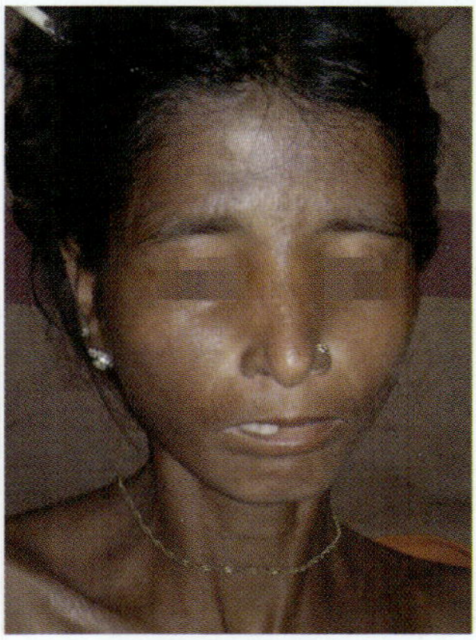

Fig. 5.39: Pigmentation in a patient of scleroderma

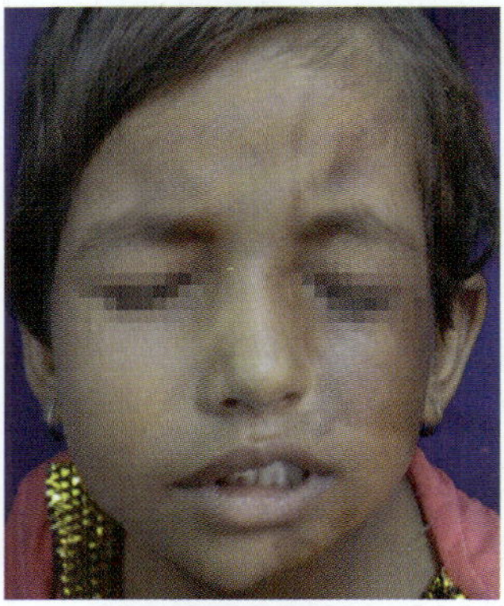

Fig. 5.40: Morphea

- Besides the pigmentation, the skin is shiny, indurated and bound down to the deeper structures.

Urticaria Pigmentosa

- Most common pattern of cutaneous mastocytosis characterized by symmetrically distributed, numerous hyperpigmented macules on trunk (Fig. 5.41) and thighs, which typically urticate upon stroking (Darier's sign).

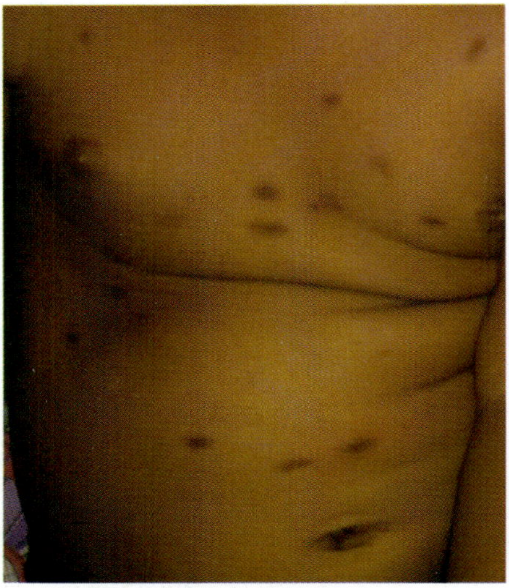

Fig. 5.41: Urticaria pigmentosa

- Usually develop in the first year of life and gradually fade away with age.

Pigmented Purpuric Dermatoses (PPD)

- A common benign condition due to capillaritis of unknown origin, presenting as asymptomatic, symmetrical, discrete to confluent, small hyperpigmented macules on legs and feet (Fig. 5.42).
- May be preceded by purpuric lesions.
- The lesions are very persistent and refractory to treatment. In most cases, only counseling suffices.

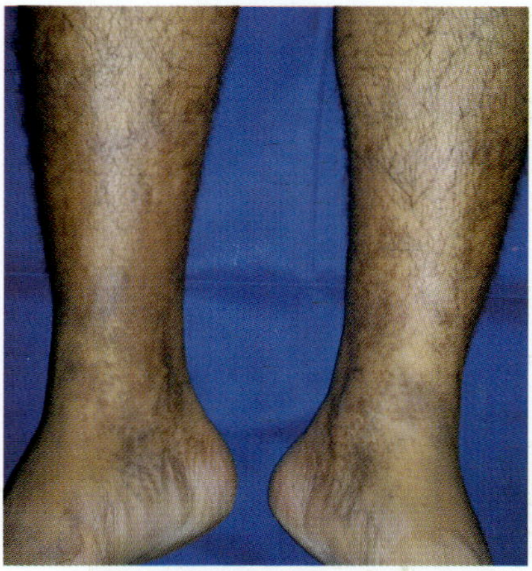

Fig. 5.42: Pigmented purpuric dermatosis on feet and legs

Erythrasma

Caused due to diphtheroids–*Corynebacterium minutissimum,* and characterized by asymptomatic, symmetrical, reddish brown/rust colored macules in flexures, most commonly axillae (Fig. 5.43). The lesions fluoresce with coral red color under Wood's light.

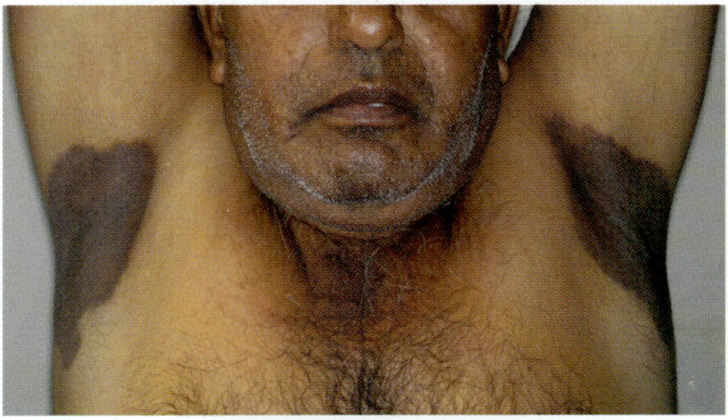

Fig. 5.43: Erythrasma

Porphyria Cutanea Tarda

A metabolic condition due to defect in heme synthesis resulting in accumulation of porphyrins. Besides pigmentation of the sun exposed skin, patients also have photosensitivity, hypertrichosis, pseudoscleroderma, increased fragility, bullae and scarring (Fig. 5.44). Urine shows reddish discoloration.

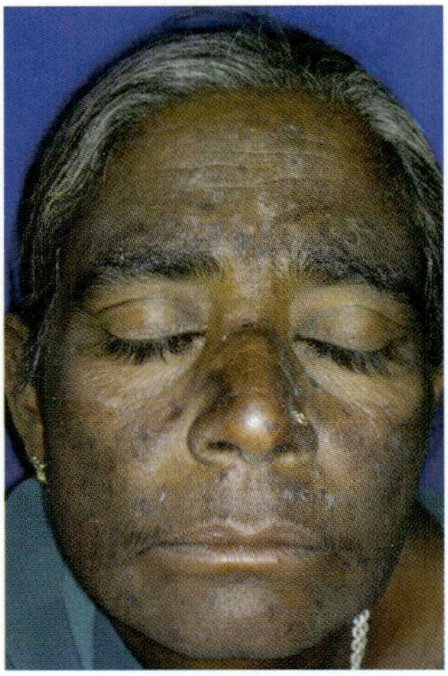

Fig. 5.44: Pigmentation in a patient of porphyria cutanea tarda

Pityriasis Versicolor

A very common, superficial fungal infection caused by *Malassezia furfur,* characterized by asymptomatic or mildly itchy, slightly scaly, hypo and hyperpigmentary macules typically over shoulders, arms, upper trunk and neck (Fig. 5.45).

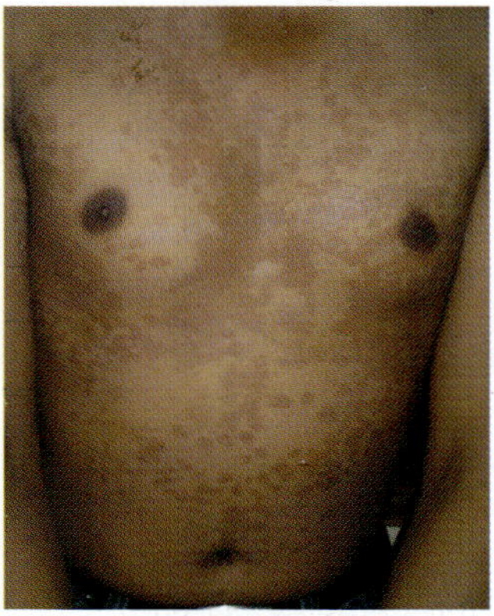

Fig. 5.45: Pityriasis versicolor

TREATMENT OF HYPERPIGMENTARY DISORDERS

- Management primarily depends on establishing and if possible, reversing/eliminating the cause.
- In patients with PIH (which usually resolves with time), non-responsive conditions and/or lesions at cosmetically insignificant sites, counseling may be all that is required/can be offered.
- In photo exposed sites, broad spectrum sunscreens should be prescribed, because sunlight intensifies the pigmentation.
- Determining the depth of pigmentation (epidermal or dermal) plays a key role in management with regard to the treatment options and expected outcome.
- Various topical depigmenting agents (e.g. Hydroquinone, arbutin, kojic acid, azelaic acid etc), peels (e.g. glycolic acid, trichloroacetic acid, Jessner's etc), and lasers (Q switched Nd: YAG, fractional etc.) can be used, either alone or in combination, with variable efficacy (for details, Chapter 4).

Suggested Readings

1. Chang MW; *Disorders of Hyperpigmentation,* In: Bolognia JL, Jorizzo JL, Schaffer JV, eds.; *Dermatology,* 3rd edn., Elsevier Saunders 2009, pp.1049-74.
2. Anstey AV; *Disorders of Skin Colour,* In: Burns T, Breathnach S, C Neil, Griffiths C, eds.; *Rook's Textbook of Dermatology,* 8th edn., West Sussex, UK: Wiley-Blackwell 2010, pp. 58.10-58.38.
3. Dhar S, Dutta P, Malakar R; *Pigmentary Disorders,* In: Valia RG, Valia AR, eds.; *IADVL Textbook of Dermatology*, 3rd edn., Mumbai: Bhalani Publishing House 2008, pp. 760-91.
4. Lahiri K, Chatterjee M, Sarkar R, eds.; *Pigmentary Disorders, A Comprehensive Compendium,* New Delhi: Jaypee Brothers Medical Publishers (P) Ltd., 2014.
5. Khanna N, Rasool S; *Facial Melanoses: Indian Perspective*; *Indian J Dermatol Venereol Leprol* 2011;77: pp. 552-64.
6. *Disorders of Hyperpigmentation*; Bolognia JL, Schaffer JV, Duncan KO, Ko CJ, eds.; *Dermatology Essentials,* New Delhi: Elsevier Saunders 2014, pp. 496-514.
7. Sardana K, Mahajan S, Jain A; *Pigmentation Disorders,* In: Sardana K, Garg VK, Mahajan S, eds.; *Diagnosis and Management of Skin Disorders. An Evidence-Based Approach,* New Delhi, Wolters Kluwer Pvt. Ltd. 2012, pp. 609-31.

INDEX

S

T

U

V

W

X

Z